Menopause Made Easy

Your Roadmap for the Menopause Journey ! Shine in Relationships, Manage Hormonal Changes and Hot Flashes, Protect Physical and Mental Health and Stay Fit with the Menopause Diet

By Victoria Hart

Table of Contents

HERE IS YOUR FREE BONUS:

Exclusive Menopause Diet with Recipes

Improve your health and well-being during menopause with our specially designed diet plan aimed at helping you lose weight and stay fit.

This expert-crafted diet is designed to support your weight management and overall fitness.

This valuable tool, available for immediate free download, is your key to maintaining health and vitality throughout your menopause journey

CLICK HERE TO DOWNLOAD IT

OR

SCAN THE QR CODE TO DOWNLOAD IT

Preface

Welcome to "Menopause Made Easy," a comprehensive guide designed to help you navigate one of life's most significant transitions with confidence and ease. Menopause is a natural part of aging, yet it often arrives with a host of questions and concerns. For many, it is a time of profound physical, emotional, and psychological changes. This book aims to demystify menopause, providing clear, concise, and practical information to support you through every stage of this journey.

We begin by discussing what menopause truly is and the transformations it brings to the menstrual cycle. Understanding these basic concepts will help you recognize and embrace the natural changes your body is experiencing. Knowledge is power, and by equipping yourself with accurate information, you can approach menopause with a sense of preparedness and calm.

Next, we delve into the myriad physical and emotional symptoms associated with menopause. From the infamous hot flashes and night sweats to mood swings and anxiety, we cover a wide range of experiences. These symptoms can often feel overwhelming, but our goal is to normalize them and offer strategies to manage them effectively. By addressing both the physical and emotional aspects, we hope to provide a holistic approach to your well-being.

Managing menopausal symptoms is a central theme throughout this book. We explore various treatment options, including hormone replacement therapy (HRT), non-hormonal treatments, and alternative and complementary therapies. Each approach has its own set of benefits and considerations, and we aim to present a balanced view to help you make informed decisions about your health care. Understanding your options allows you to tailor a treatment plan that best suits your individual needs.

Long-term health and wellness are vital during and after menopause. Maintaining bone health, preventing osteoporosis, ensuring cardiovascular health, and nurturing sexual health and intimacy are crucial for a vibrant and fulfilling life beyond menopause. By taking proactive steps now, you can lay the groundwork for a healthier future.

We also offer practical advice and lifestyle adjustments to enhance your overall well-being. Topics such as diet and nutrition, exercise and fitness, and sleep and relaxation are covered in detail. Small, manageable changes can have a significant impact, and we provide actionable tips to incorporate into your daily routine. Your lifestyle choices play a crucial role in how you experience menopause, and we are here to guide you in making positive changes.

Emotional and social well-being are equally important. We discuss mental health and cognitive function, the importance of building support networks, and strategies for empowerment and self-care. This book emphasizes the holistic nature of health, highlighting the interconnectedness of physical, emotional, and social factors.

Maintaining strong social connections and seeking support can significantly enhance your quality of life.

We have included a treasure trove of resources and further reading. You will find expert interviews and case studies, useful tools and resources, and answers to frequently asked questions and common concerns. This section serves as a valuable reference, offering deeper insights and practical solutions to everyday challenges.

Finally, the appendices provide additional context and support for the topics discussed throughout the book. A glossary of terms, a reference list citing studies and articles, and a detailed index make it easy to navigate and find the information you need.

"Menopause Made Easy" is more than just a book; it is a companion on your journey through menopause. We hope that the information, insights, and encouragement within these pages will help you embrace this phase of life with grace and resilience. Welcome to your guide to making menopause easier and more manageable.

CHAPTER 1

THE MENOPAUSE

Introduction

The Journey of Menopause: An Overview

Menopause stands as a pivotal chapter in the narrative of a woman's life, signaling the sunset of her reproductive era. This natural biological progression gracefully unfolds, typically straddling the years between 45 and 55, though its onset may vary, introducing itself earlier or later in some. Navigating this transformative phase with knowledge and grace is paramount in mastering its myriad symptoms and welcoming the evolution it ushers in. As we delve into the nuances of menopause, it becomes essential to understand its impacts not just on the body, but on the psyche and overall life of a woman, transforming a seemingly challenging time into a period of rejuvenation and empowerment.

The Phases of Menopause

Perimenopause: The Transition Begins

Perimenopause marks the elegant prelude to menopause, often making its entrance in a woman's 40s, though it can debut in the 30s. During this transitional phase, the ovaries subtly reduce estrogen production, leading to enchanting fluctuations in hormone levels. Spanning several years, perimenopause is defined by its hallmark of irregular menstrual cycles. Women may encounter a spectrum of symptoms, including hot flashes, night sweats, mood swings, and shifts in libido. This period of profound hormonal upheaval is pivotal, and a deep understanding of these changes can empower women, allowing them to gracefully embrace the forthcoming chapter of menopause.

Menopause: The Official Milestone

Menopause is elegantly confirmed when a woman has not experienced a menstrual period for 12 consecutive months. At this sophisticated juncture, the ovaries have ceased their enchanting release of eggs, and estrogen levels have dramatically waned. The average age for this grand transition is 51, though it can vary across the spectrum of womanhood. During this stage, one might encounter the likes of hot flashes, vaginal dryness, sleep disturbances, and weight gain. These symptoms, ranging from the subtle to the intense, weave their impact on daily life, adding yet another layer to the complex and beautiful tapestry of a woman's journey. daily life and overall well-being. Recognizing menopause as a natural and inevitable phase can help women approach it with a proactive and positive mindset.

Post-menopause: Life After Menstruation

Post-menopause marks a new chapter, a refined stage following menopause that graces a woman for the rest of her life. In this era, the intensity of hot flashes and night sweats may gracefully wane for many. Yet, the lower levels of estrogen usher in an increased risk for certain health concerns, notably osteoporosis and cardiovascular disease. Prioritizing long-term health and preventive care becomes paramount during this sophisticated phase. Regular check-ups, a meticulously balanced diet, and a vibrant, active lifestyle are essential to maintaining overall health and enhancing the quality of life. Embrace this stage with elegance and care, ensuring that wellness remains at the forefront of your journey.

The Emotional and Psychological Impact

The journey of menopause transcends the physical, elegantly intertwining emotional and psychological transitions. Hormonal fluctuations can evoke mood swings, anxiety, and even bouts of depression. For some, the cessation of menstruation may stir a poignant sense of loss, while others might find solace in the newfound freedom. It's vital to acknowledge and embrace these emotions, seeking support as needed. Cultivating open dialogue with family, friends, and healthcare providers offers not only emotional solace but also invaluable practical advice. In this transformative phase, let understanding and communication be your chic allies, ensuring you navigate with grace and confidence.

Navigating the Journey

Every woman's menopause journey is a distinctive experience, requiring a tailored approach. Here are some chic strategies to navigate this transformative phase:

Educate Yourself: Knowledge is power. Understanding the biological processes and symptoms of menopause empowers you to make informed health decisions.

Seek Medical Advice: Regular consultations with your healthcare provider can help manage symptoms and monitor health risks. Explore options like hormone replacement therapy (HRT) and other treatments if necessary.

Adopt a Healthy Lifestyle: Elevate your well-being with a balanced diet, regular exercise, and stress management techniques. These lifestyle adjustments can significantly alleviate symptoms and enhance overall wellness.

Build a Support System: Connect with other fabulous women navigating menopause, join support groups, and share experiences. Emotional support is a game-changer.

Embrace the Change: View menopause as a new, empowering chapter. Focus on the positive aspects, such as freedom from menstruation and the opportunity to prioritize your personal health and well-being.

In conclusion, the menopause journey is a multifaceted experience that encompasses physical, emotional, and psychological changes. By understanding the phases and impacts of menopause, women can navigate this transition with confidence and grace, embracing the vibrant new phase of life it brings.

Why This Book? Addressing Common Concerns and Misconceptions

Menopause, a natural phase in every woman's life, often remains cloaked in myths, misconceptions, and misunderstandings. Many women approach this stage with a cocktail of fear, confusion, and misinformation, intensifying their symptoms and piling on unnecessary stress. This book is your chic guide to demystifying menopause, addressing common concerns and debunking misconceptions, while providing you with the knowledge and tools to navigate this transition with unparalleled confidence and ease. Let's embrace this transformative journey with sophistication and grace.

Understanding Menopause: Breaking the Silence

One of the most pressing issues surrounding menopause is the stark absence of open dialogue. Traditionally, menopause has been a hush-hush topic, relegated to whispered conversations behind closed doors or brushed off as an inevitable byproduct of aging. This silence has cultivated a myriad of myths and misconceptions.

By illuminating menopause in this book, we aim to elevate the conversation, empowering women to share their experiences with confidence, sans shame or embarrassment. It's time to break the silence and embrace this natural phase with sophistication and pride.

Menopause Means the End of Youth and Vitality

A prevalent misconception is that menopause signals the end of a woman's youth and vitality. Many women fear that they will become invisible, irrelevant, or less feminine. This book dispels this myth by emphasizing that menopause is not an end but a transition. It is an opportunity to embrace a new phase of life, often with increased wisdom, self-assurance, and freedom from the constraints of menstruation and fertility concerns. Menopause can be a time of renewal and rediscovery, where women can focus on their passions, health, and well-being with a newfound perspective.

Menopause Symptoms Are the Same for Everyone

Another common misconception is that all women experience menopause in the same way. In reality, menopause is a highly individualized experience. Symptoms vary widely in type, severity, and duration. This book provides a comprehensive overview of possible symptoms, from hot flashes and night sweats to mood swings and cognitive changes, while emphasizing that each woman's journey is unique. It encourages women to listen to their bodies and seek personalized medical advice, highlighting the importance of understanding one's own unique experience and managing it in the best way possible.

Hormone Replacement Therapy (HRT) Is Dangerous

There is significant controversy and confusion surrounding Hormone Replacement Therapy (HRT). Many women fear that HRT is inherently dangerous and should be avoided at all costs.

This book addresses the benefits and risks of HRT based on the latest scientific research. It provides balanced information, helping women make informed decisions in consultation with their healthcare providers. The book also explores alternative treatments and lifestyle changes that can help manage symptoms. By presenting a clear, evidence-based perspective, this book aims to dispel the fears and myths surrounding HRT, allowing women to make choices that are best suited for their health and lifestyle.

Menopause Only Affects Physical Health

While physical symptoms are often the most discussed aspect of menopause, the emotional and psychological impacts are equally important. Many women experience mood swings, anxiety, depression, and cognitive changes. This book delves into the emotional landscape of menopause, offering strategies for mental well-being and emphasizing the importance of holistic health. It encourages women to seek support from loved ones, mental health professionals, and support groups. Understanding that menopause affects both the body and the mind is crucial for comprehensive care, and this book aims to provide the tools and resources needed for overall well-being during this transition.

Empowerment Through Knowledge

This book is your ultimate guide, seamlessly blending scientific insights with practical advice and heartfelt personal stories. It's crafted to empower women with clear, accurate, and compassionate information. By tackling common concerns and debunking misconceptions, this book aims to transform fear and confusion into confidence and clarity. It inspires women to take charge of their health and well-being, encouraging them to ask questions, seek support, and embrace menopause as a natural, enriching phase of life.

In essence, this book goes beyond merely managing menopause; it's a rallying cry to break the silence, shatter myths, and empower women. It stands as a supportive and enlightening resource, guiding women through the complexities of menopause and helping them flourish during this pivotal life transition.

What Is Menopause?

Definitions and Phases: Perimenopause, Menopause, and Post-menopause

Understanding the journey through menopause requires clarity on its three distinct phases: perimenopause, menopause, and post-menopause. Each stage comes with its own set of symptoms, challenges, and transformations, marking significant shifts in a woman's reproductive life. By defining and elaborating on these phases, women can better navigate the changes they experience and seek appropriate care and support.

Perimenopause, meaning "around menopause," is the transitional period leading up to menopause. It typically begins in a woman's 40s but can start as early as her mid-30s. This phase can last anywhere from a few years to over a decade, ending only when menopause is reached.

During perimenopause, the ovaries gradually produce less estrogen, causing hormonal fluctuations that lead to various symptoms. Common signs include irregular menstrual cycles, hot flashes, night sweats, mood swings, sleep disturbances, and changes in libido. Women may also experience physical changes like weight gain, especially around the abdomen, and alterations in skin texture and hair.

One hallmark of perimenopause is the unpredictability of menstrual cycles. Periods may become erratic—sometimes shorter, sometimes longer, heavier or lighter, and more or less frequent. These irregularities are due to the erratic nature of ovarian function during this stage.

Understanding perimenopause is crucial because it prepares women for the eventual transition to menopause. Recognizing the symptoms and changes can prompt timely discussions with healthcare providers, leading to better symptom management and overall health.

Menopause is officially defined as the point in time when a woman has not had a menstrual period for 12 consecutive months. The average age of menopause is 51, but it can occur earlier or later.

This stage marks the end of a woman's reproductive years as the ovaries cease to release eggs and produce significant amounts of estrogen and progesterone.

The symptoms experienced during menopause are often a continuation of those from perimenopause but may vary in intensity. Hot flashes, night sweats, and vaginal dryness are among the most common complaints. These symptoms can significantly impact a woman's quality of life, affecting sleep, mood, and overall well-being.

Menopause also brings an increased risk of certain health conditions due to lower estrogen levels. These include osteoporosis, cardiovascular disease, and changes in metabolism. It is essential for women to monitor their health closely during this time and adopt lifestyle changes that support long-term well-being.

Post-menopause refers to the years following menopause, starting from the 12-month mark after the last menstrual period. During post-menopause, many of the symptoms experienced during perimenopause and menopause gradually diminish, although some women may continue to experience them for a longer duration.

The primary concern in post-menopause is managing long-term health risks associated with reduced estrogen levels. Osteoporosis becomes a significant risk due to decreased bone density, making fractures more likely. Heart health is another critical area, as the protective effects of estrogen on the cardiovascular system wane.

Women in post-menopause should focus on maintaining a healthy lifestyle, including a balanced diet rich in calcium and vitamin D, regular weight-bearing exercise, and routine health screenings. Hormone replacement therapy (HRT) may be considered for some women to alleviate persistent symptoms and reduce health risks, but it should be discussed thoroughly with a healthcare provider to weigh the benefits and potential risks.

Navigating through perimenopause, menopause, and post-menopause involves understanding the unique characteristics and challenges of each phase. By defining these stages and recognizing the symptoms and health implications associated with them, women can better prepare for and manage this significant transition. This knowledge empowers women to take proactive steps in maintaining their health and well-being throughout their menopausal journey and beyond.

Definitions and Phases: Biological and Hormonal Changes

Menopause heralds a transformative chapter in a woman's life, characterized by a cascade of biological and hormonal changes that redefine her physiology. This multifaceted journey spans several years, and each phase brings its unique set of challenges and revelations. Understanding these intricate transformations empowers women to navigate menopause with sophistication and insight.

At the core of menopause lies the dramatic shift in hormonal dynamics that orchestrates a woman's reproductive system. The primary hormones, estrogen and progesterone, which are synthesized by the ovaries, play pivotal roles throughout this transition.

Perimenopause, often described as a hormonal rollercoaster, marks the beginning of this journey. During this stage, estrogen levels start to fluctuate unpredictably, deviating from the regular menstrual cycle's orderly pattern. These erratic estrogen surges and drops are the culprits behind many hallmark symptoms of perimenopause, such as hot flashes, mood swings, and irregular menstrual cycles. Concurrently, progesterone levels begin their gradual decline, which can result in longer, heavier periods, contributing to the cycle irregularities experienced by many women.

As a woman transitions into menopause, these hormonal shifts reach a climax. Menopause is defined by the cessation of menstrual periods for 12 consecutive months, signaling the ovaries' dramatic reduction in estrogen and progesterone production. This decline heralds the end of reproductive capability and ushers in symptoms like vaginal dryness, hot flashes, and night sweats. Additionally, the pituitary gland's response to dropping estrogen levels by increasing Follicle-Stimulating Hormone (FSH) production serves as a biological marker for menopause, detectable through blood tests.

Post-menopause, the final stage, sees hormone levels stabilizing at a persistently low level. While many acute menopausal symptoms may subside, the enduring impact of reduced estrogen becomes more pronounced. This stage brings heightened risks for conditions such as osteoporosis and cardiovascular diseases due to the sustained low estrogen levels. The complete cessation of progesterone further affects various bodily systems, particularly those associated with reproductive and sexual health.

The biological repercussions of these hormonal upheavals are extensive, influencing everything from bone density to cardiovascular health. A critical concern is the reduction in bone density, as estrogen is vital for maintaining bone strength. Its decline accelerates bone resorption, increasing the likelihood of osteoporosis, characterized by brittle and fragile bones prone to fractures.

Cardiovascular health also takes a hit post-menopause. Estrogen's protective effects on the heart, such as promoting good cholesterol (HDL) and reducing bad cholesterol (LDL), diminish, elevating the risk of heart disease and stroke. Metabolic changes are another significant aspect, with hormonal shifts often leading to slower metabolism and subsequent weight gain, particularly around the abdomen. This central adiposity is linked to heightened risks for diabetes and metabolic syndrome. Additionally, the body's handling of insulin can be impaired, increasing the susceptibility to insulin resistance and type 2 diabetes.

Urogenital changes further compound the challenges. The drop in estrogen levels can cause vaginal atrophy, leading to thinning, dryness, and inflammation of the vaginal walls. This results in discomfort, urinary incontinence, and painful intercourse. Moreover, the pelvic floor muscles may weaken, exacerbating urinary incontinence and other pelvic floor disorders.

Cognitive and emotional health are also significantly influenced by menopause. Estrogen is believed to have neuroprotective effects, and its decline can affect brain function, potentially increasing the risk of neurodegenerative diseases like Alzheimer's. Hormonal fluctuations can impact neurotransmitters, leading to mood swings, anxiety, and depression.

Understanding the biological and hormonal changes during menopause is crucial for anticipating and managing the symptoms that accompany this transition. This knowledge empowers women to take proactive steps in preserving their health and well-being. Seeking medical advice and support is essential in navigating menopause with confidence and grace, ensuring that this phase of life is not just a transition but a period of renewal and empowerment.

The Menstrual Cycle
And Its Changes

How Menstrual Patterns Alter Leading to Menopause

Menopause represents a pivotal chapter in a woman's life, ushering in the cessation of menstrual cycles and signaling the close of her reproductive years. This transition is not abrupt; it unfolds gradually, manifesting through noticeable shifts in menstrual patterns. Gaining a clear understanding of these changes empowers women to anticipate what lies ahead and recognize the signs heralding menopause.

Perimenopause, the precursor to menopause, typically spans several years before menstruation halts entirely. This phase often commences in the early 40s, though it can begin as early as the late 30s. During perimenopause, women observe significant alterations in their menstrual cycles, an early indicator of the body's evolving hormonal landscape.

One of the hallmark signs of perimenopause is irregular periods. A woman who has previously enjoyed a consistent 28-day cycle may suddenly find her periods occurring 21 days apart one month and 35 days the next. This irregularity stems from the ovaries' erratic function, disrupting the hormone levels that regulate the menstrual cycle. As a result, the predictability that once characterized her cycles gives way to a new, uncertain rhythm.

The flow of menstrual bleeding also transforms during perimenopause. Some women experience menorrhagia, where bleeding becomes notably heavier and prolonged. Conversely, others may notice a reduction in flow, with lighter and shorter periods. These fluctuations are a direct consequence of estrogen levels swinging unpredictably, either causing the uterine lining to thicken excessively or shed more sporadically.

As menopause draws nearer, missed periods become more frequent. Women might go several months without menstruating, only for their period to return unexpectedly. This sporadic pattern is due to the ovaries' diminishing ability to ovulate consistently, resulting in erratic hormone production.

Spotting or light bleeding between periods is another common occurrence during perimenopause.

While often harmless and indicative of hormonal shifts, persistent or heavy spotting should prompt a visit to a healthcare provider to rule out other potential conditions.

The alterations in menstrual patterns during perimenopause are primarily driven by shifts in two key hormones: estrogen and progesterone, produced by the ovaries. Estrogen levels during perimenopause can be particularly volatile, with periods of elevated estrogen followed by sharp declines. Elevated estrogen can cause heavier menstrual bleeding, whereas low estrogen might lead to missed periods or lighter flows. Concurrently, the decline in progesterone, which regulates the menstrual cycle and supports pregnancy, contributes to the irregularity of periods and can lead to prolonged, heavier bleeding when ovulation is inconsistent.

Menopause itself is diagnosed when a woman has not had a menstrual period for 12 consecutive months. The average age for menopause is around 51, though it can vary. The final menstrual period, or FMP, is identified retrospectively, confirmed only after a year without periods. The time leading up to this milestone is marked by increased menstrual irregularity, signifying the body's transition.

Following the FMP, women enter the postmenopausal phase. During this stage, the ovaries produce minimal estrogen and progesterone. Menstrual bleeding ceases entirely, and the body adapts to its new hormonal norm.

Understanding the changes in menstrual patterns leading up to menopause is crucial for recognizing the signs of this significant life stage. Women are encouraged to track their menstrual cycles to detect emerging trends and shifts over time. Open communication with healthcare providers about any notable changes or concerns is essential for effectively managing symptoms and maintaining overall health during this transition.

In summary, the journey to menopause encompasses various changes in menstrual patterns driven by hormonal fluctuations. From irregular periods and altered flow to missed periods and spotting, these changes, while normal, require awareness and proactive management. Recognizing these shifts enables women to approach the transition to menopause with confidence and clarity, embracing this natural phase of life.

Understanding Irregular Periods and Their Implications

Irregular periods are a hallmark of the transitional phase known as perimenopause, leading up to menopause. This phase can span several years and involves significant changes in menstrual patterns due to fluctuating hormone levels. Understanding these irregularities and their implications is crucial for women navigating this life stage with confidence and grace.

What Constitutes Irregular Periods?

Irregular periods during perimenopause manifest in various ways. A menstrual cycle is considered irregular when the length varies significantly from month to month. For instance, if the cycle length fluctuates widely or if periods are missed altogether, this is termed irregular.

Variations in Cycle Length:

Normal menstrual cycles typically range from 21 to 35 days. During perimenopause, these cycles can become shorter (less than 21 days) or longer (more than 35 days). This inconsistency is one of the most noticeable changes women may experience, creating an unpredictable rhythm that can be challenging to manage.

Changes in Flow:

Women may notice variations in the flow of their periods. Some may experience unusually heavy periods, known as menorrhagia, while others may have very light bleeding, termed

hypomenorrhea. The duration of bleeding can also change, becoming either shorter or longer than usual, adding another layer of unpredictability.

Missed Periods:

Skipped periods are a common occurrence during perimenopause. A woman might miss several months of periods and then suddenly have a normal cycle. This irregularity can create uncertainty and concern, as the body's usual cycle becomes increasingly erratic.

Spotting Between Periods:

Some women may experience spotting or light bleeding between regular periods. This can be due to hormonal imbalances affecting the endometrial lining of the uterus, further complicating the menstrual pattern and adding to the anxiety around menstrual health.

Hormonal Causes of Irregular Periods

The primary drivers of irregular periods during perimenopause are changes in the levels of estrogen and progesterone. These hormones regulate the menstrual cycle, and their fluctuating levels lead to the irregularities experienced.

Estrogen Fluctuations:

Estrogen levels can become erratic, leading to cycles where the uterine lining builds up more than usual, resulting in heavier periods. Conversely, lower levels of estrogen can cause lighter periods or missed cycles, contributing to the unpredictability.

Progesterone Decline:

Progesterone, produced after ovulation, helps stabilize the uterine lining. As ovulation becomes irregular, progesterone levels decline, contributing to unpredictable menstrual patterns and creating a cascade of changes that affect overall health.

Implications of Irregular Periods

Irregular periods, while often a normal part of the perimenopausal transition, can have various implications for a woman's health and well-being.

Physical Health:

Heavy bleeding can lead to anemia, characterized by fatigue, weakness, and dizziness. Women experiencing unusually heavy periods should consult a healthcare provider to manage these symptoms effectively and ensure they maintain optimal health.

Emotional and Psychological Impact:

The unpredictability of periods can cause significant stress and anxiety. Women may feel unprepared for sudden heavy bleeding or become anxious about the uncertainty of their cycles, impacting their emotional and psychological well-being.

Impact on Daily Life:

Irregular periods can interfere with daily activities and lifestyle. Planning around an unpredictable menstrual cycle can be challenging, affecting work, social life, and physical activities, necessitating a flexible and adaptive approach to daily living.

Need for Medical Evaluation:

While irregular periods are common during perimenopause, they can sometimes indicate other health issues, such as thyroid problems, fibroids, or polyps. It is important for women to seek medical evaluation to rule out these conditions and ensure their health is not compromised.

Managing Irregular Periods

There are several strategies to manage the symptoms and implications of irregular periods.

Lifestyle Adjustments:

Maintaining a healthy lifestyle with regular exercise and a balanced diet can help manage symptoms. Stress reduction techniques such as yoga and meditation can also be beneficial in maintaining overall well-being.

Medical Treatments:

Hormone therapy or birth control pills can help regulate menstrual cycles. Other medications may be prescribed to manage heavy bleeding or other symptoms, providing relief and stability during this transition.

Regular Monitoring:

Keeping track of menstrual cycles can help women understand their patterns and anticipate changes. Apps and calendars can be useful tools for tracking, allowing for better preparation and management.

Consulting Healthcare Providers:

Regular check-ups with a healthcare provider can ensure that any underlying issues are addressed promptly and that appropriate treatment strategies are in place, ensuring comprehensive care and support.

Understanding irregular periods and their implications is essential for women approaching menopause. Recognizing that these changes are a normal part of the perimenopausal transition can help alleviate anxiety and ensure that women seek appropriate care and support to manage their symptoms effectively, embracing this natural phase of life with confidence.

CHAPTER 2

Physical And Emotional Symptoms

Common Physical Symptoms

Hot Flashes and Night Sweats

Hot flashes and night sweats are the quintessential companions on the tumultuous journey through menopause. These vasomotor symptoms, driven by shifting hormone levels—especially the decline in estrogen—disrupt the body's thermostat, leading to waves of heat that can feel like an uninvited guest at the chicest soirée. Understanding the essence of these hot flashes and night sweats, their profound impact on daily life, and the myriad ways to manage them, is key for women navigating this transformative phase.

Picture this: hot flashes are sudden, fiery bursts of heat that blaze across the face, neck, and chest, often leaving a trail of redness and sweat in their wake. They strike without warning, lasting anywhere from a fleeting moment to several minutes. The frequency and intensity vary widely among women; some may encounter them sporadically, while others face them with relentless regularity. Night sweats, essentially hot flashes that invade your sleep, are the nocturnal tormentors that disrupt rest and leave you battling fatigue.

The science behind these heat waves? It's all about the hypothalamus, the brain's temperature-control center. When estrogen levels plummet, the hypothalamus becomes overly sensitive to even the slightest temperature changes. This hyper-sensitivity prompts the body to overreact to minor fluctuations, sparking a hot flash. Blood vessels near the skin's surface dilate, releasing heat and bringing on that unmistakable flush of warmth and sweat.

The daily impact of hot flashes and night sweats can be nothing short of dramatic. By day, these episodes can be a cocktail of discomfort and embarrassment, especially in social or professional settings. Women often feel the sting of self-consciousness as they battle visible sweat or a sudden flush. These interruptions can shatter concentration and derail productivity, turning routine tasks into monumental challenges. At night, the relentless wake-ups caused by night sweats wreak havoc on sleep quality, leading to daytime fatigue, irritability, and a struggle to focus, diminishing overall well-being.

Managing these symptoms often requires a sophisticated blend of lifestyle tweaks, non-hormonal treatments, and, at times, hormone therapy. Starting with lifestyle changes, these are your first-line defense and can be remarkably effective. Staying cool with layers, fans, and a perfectly balanced room temperature can tame the intensity of hot flashes. Steering clear of triggers like spicy foods, caffeine, alcohol, and stress can also help curb their frequency. Regular exercise and maintaining a healthy weight have proven to be powerful allies in alleviating symptoms for many women.

Non-hormonal options are diverse and include medications like selective serotonin reuptake inhibitors (SSRIs) and gabapentin, which have been shown to diminish the frequency and severity of hot flashes. These treatments are a godsend for those who cannot or prefer not to opt for hormone therapy. Herbal supplements, including black cohosh and soy isoflavones, are popular natural remedies, though their effectiveness can be hit or miss, so a chat with a healthcare provider is essential.

Hormone therapy, with estrogen or a combo of estrogen and progesterone, remains a gold standard in tackling hot flashes and night sweats. Yet, it's typically advised for the shortest duration possible due to potential risks like increased breast cancer, heart disease, and stroke. Women contemplating hormone therapy should engage in a thorough discussion with their healthcare provider, weighing the benefits and risks tailored to their health profile and symptom severity.

In essence, hot flashes and night sweats are signature symptoms of menopause, casting a significant shadow over a woman's daily life and well-being. Grasping their origins, effects, and management strategies is crucial for navigating this complex phase with grace. By blending lifestyle adjustments, non-hormonal treatments, and thoughtful consideration of hormone therapy, women can find the relief they seek, enhancing their quality of life through the menopausal journey.

Vaginal Dryness and Discomfort

Vaginal dryness and discomfort—two uninvited guests that often accompany the grand transition of menopause. These distressing symptoms are primarily the result of a decline in estrogen levels, a hormone vital for maintaining the health, elasticity, and natural lubrication of vaginal tissues. As estrogen bids its farewell, the vaginal walls thin, lose their supple elasticity, and become drier, ushering in a cascade of discomfort, irritation, and pain.

The transformation in vaginal health during menopause can cast a shadow over a woman's quality of life, impacting not just physical comfort but also emotional well-being and intimate relationships. Persistent itching and burning sensations become daily companions, turning even the simplest activities such as sitting, walking, or exercising into uncomfortable endeavors. This constant awareness and discomfort can diminish the enjoyment of daily life and erode overall happiness.

Sexual intercourse can become a painful ordeal due to the lack of natural lubrication, a condition known as dyspareunia. This pain can lead to a reduction in sexual desire and an avoidance of intimacy, potentially straining relationships. Many women, feeling embarrassed or reluctant to discuss these intimate issues, may isolate themselves, exacerbating feelings of frustration and loneliness.

Addressing vaginal dryness and discomfort calls for a multi-faceted approach, combining self-care strategies, over-the-counter remedies, and medical treatments. Vaginal moisturizers and lubricants stand at the forefront of self-care solutions. Regular use of vaginal moisturizers helps maintain moisture and elasticity in the vaginal tissues, mimicking the natural secretions that keep the area hydrated and comfortable. During sexual activity, lubricants can reduce friction and discomfort, available in water-based, silicone-based, or oil-based formulas to suit individual preferences and sensitivities.

For more persistent or severe symptoms, medical treatments may be necessary. Local estrogen therapy, directly applied to the vaginal area via creams, tablets, or rings, can work wonders. This treatment restores the health of vaginal tissues, boosts natural lubrication, and alleviates discomfort without significantly altering overall hormone levels. By targeting the problem area directly, this approach minimizes the risks associated with systemic hormone replacement therapy.

Additionally, non-hormonal prescription medications like prasterone (DHEA) and ospemifene have emerged as effective treatments for vaginal dryness and discomfort. These medications target the root causes of vaginal atrophy and dryness, enhancing tissue health and reducing symptoms.

Lifestyle changes also play a pivotal role in managing vaginal dryness and discomfort. Staying hydrated, consuming a balanced diet rich in omega-3 fatty acids, and avoiding irritants such as harsh soaps, douches, and synthetic underwear can help maintain vaginal health. Regular sexual activity, including non-penetrative intimacy, promotes blood flow to the vaginal area, supporting tissue health and vitality.

Emotional support and open communication are essential in managing the impact of vaginal dryness on relationships. Encouraging candid conversations with partners about these issues fosters understanding and intimacy, lightening the emotional load of these physical changes. Seeking support from healthcare providers, counselors, or support groups can provide valuable resources and reassurance.

In essence, vaginal dryness and discomfort present significant challenges during menopause, affecting physical comfort, emotional well-being, and intimate relationships. By employing a combination of self-care strategies, over-the-counter remedies, medical treatments, and open communication, women can effectively manage these symptoms and enhance their quality of life during this transformative period. Addressing this issue with sensitivity and understanding is crucial, recognizing its profound impact on a woman's overall health and happiness.

Sleep Disturbances and Fatigue

Sleep disturbances and fatigue are among the most pervasive and disruptive symptoms that women encounter during menopause, casting a long shadow over daily life, overall well-being, and quality of life. Navigating this transitional phase with elegance and grace begins with understanding the root causes, impacts, and management strategies of these challenges.

Menopausal hormonal fluctuations lie at the heart of sleep disturbances. The decline in estrogen and progesterone levels directly influences sleep regulation. Estrogen plays a pivotal role in ensuring time spent in deep sleep, the most restorative phase of the sleep cycle. As estrogen levels fall, many women find themselves waking frequently throughout the night, struggling to achieve a restful slumber. Progesterone, with its calming effects, also wanes during menopause, potentially heightening anxiety and making it more difficult to drift off to sleep.

Hot flashes and night sweats, quintessential hallmarks of menopause, exacerbate these sleep issues. These sudden surges of heat and subsequent sweating can jolt women awake multiple times during the night, preventing uninterrupted sleep. The discomfort and unpredictability of these episodes often lead to anticipatory anxiety, where women become anxious about the potential for sleep disruption, further complicating their ability to rest peacefully.

The cumulative result of these sleep disturbances is chronic fatigue. Women suffering from menopausal sleep issues often wake up feeling anything but refreshed, regardless of how many hours they've spent in bed. This persistent tiredness infiltrates every aspect of life, affecting work performance and personal relationships alike. Fatigue can impair cognitive functions, leading to struggles with concentration, memory, and decision-making. Moreover, it can dampen mood, heightening the risk of depression and anxiety.

Addressing sleep disturbances and fatigue during menopause requires a multifaceted approach. Establishing good sleep hygiene is foundational. This involves maintaining a consistent sleep schedule—going to bed and waking up at the same time daily—creating a serene, cool sleeping environment, and steering clear of stimulants like caffeine and electronic screens before bedtime. Regular physical activity, particularly earlier in the day, can also promote better sleep by reducing anxiety and boosting overall physical tiredness.

Managing hot flashes and night sweats can significantly enhance sleep quality. Simple strategies such as wearing lightweight, breathable clothing, using fans or air conditioning in the bedroom, and practicing relaxation techniques like deep breathing or meditation before bed can be highly effective. For some women, hormone replacement therapy (HRT) or non-hormonal medications might be necessary to control severe hot flashes and improve sleep.

Cognitive-behavioral therapy (CBT) has shown remarkable effectiveness in treating insomnia and the anxiety that often accompanies it. CBT focuses on transforming negative thought patterns and behaviors that contribute to sleep problems. By addressing the mental and emotional aspects of sleep disturbances, women can develop healthier sleep habits and reduce anxiety related to sleep.

Seeking support from healthcare providers is also crucial. A doctor can help identify any underlying medical conditions, such as sleep apnea or thyroid disorders, that might be contributing to sleep disturbances and fatigue. They can also provide guidance on the safe use of sleep aids or other treatments tailored to individual needs.

Emotional and social support are equally vital. Sharing experiences with friends, family, or support groups can alleviate feelings of isolation and offer practical coping tips. Encouraging open dialogue with partners about sleep issues can foster understanding and support within relationships.

In essence, sleep disturbances and fatigue are formidable challenges during menopause, driven by hormonal changes and exacerbated by symptoms like hot flashes. Through the adoption of good sleep hygiene practices, addressing underlying symptoms, seeking professional support, and engaging in cognitive-behavioral therapy, women can improve their sleep quality and manage fatigue more effectively. Understanding and addressing these issues can lead to an enhanced quality of life and a greater sense of well-being during the menopausal transition.

Weight Gain and Metabolism Changes

Weight gain and metabolism changes are perennial concerns for women during menopause, often adding a layer of complexity to the emotional and physical challenges of this transitional period. Embracing a sophisticated understanding of the underlying causes, coupled with effective strategies, can empower women to maintain a healthy weight and overall well-being with grace and poise.

As women approach menopause, the hormonal symphony within their bodies begins to shift, particularly marked by a decline in estrogen levels. Estrogen, a key player in regulating body weight and fat distribution, gradually diminishes, prompting the body to store more fat, especially around the abdomen. This transformation from a more even fat distribution to central obesity not only alters physical appearance but also escalates the risk of metabolic disorders, such as insulin resistance, type 2 diabetes, and cardiovascular diseases.

Another factor that contributes to weight gain during menopause is the natural age-related decrease in muscle mass, known as sarcopenia. Muscle tissue, being more metabolically active than fat tissue, burns more calories at rest. As muscle mass declines, the basal metabolic rate (BMR) decreases, leading to fewer calories burned throughout the day. Thus, even if a woman's calorie intake remains unchanged, she may start to gain weight due to this reduced calorie expenditure.

Lifestyle changes that often accompany midlife can further influence weight gain. Many women experience heightened stress levels during menopause, stemming from various sources such as career pressures, family responsibilities, and the physical and emotional symptoms of menopause itself. Elevated stress levels can lead to emotional eating and cravings for high-calorie, sugary foods. Moreover, stress triggers the release of cortisol, a hormone that promotes fat storage, particularly in the abdominal area.

Sleep disturbances, which are common during menopause, exacerbate weight gain. Poor sleep quality and insufficient rest disrupt the balance of hunger-regulating hormones, ghrelin and leptin. Ghrelin, which stimulates appetite, tends to increase, while leptin, which signals fullness, decreases. This hormonal imbalance can lead to heightened hunger and overeating, complicating the maintenance of a healthy weight.

To manage weight gain and metabolic changes during menopause, adopting a holistic approach is essential. Regular physical activity plays a crucial role in maintaining muscle mass and boosting metabolism. Strength training exercises, such as weight lifting or resistance band workouts, are particularly effective in preserving and building muscle. Incorporating aerobic exercises, such as walking, jogging, or swimming, helps burn calories and improve cardiovascular health.

Dietary adjustments are also pivotal in managing weight during menopause. A balanced diet rich in whole foods, including fruits, vegetables, lean proteins, and healthy fats, supports overall health and weight management. Reducing the intake of processed foods, sugary snacks, and high-fat meals helps prevent excess calorie consumption. Paying attention to portion sizes and practicing mindful eating can also prevent overeating.

Managing stress through relaxation techniques, such as yoga, meditation, or deep breathing exercises, reduces the likelihood of emotional eating. Establishing a consistent sleep routine and creating a conducive sleep environment can improve sleep quality and support weight management efforts. Consulting a healthcare provider or a registered dietitian offers personalized guidance and support for weight management during menopause.

Weight gain and metabolism changes during menopause are influenced by hormonal fluctuations, decreased muscle mass, lifestyle factors, and stress. Understanding these elements and implementing strategies such as regular exercise, a balanced diet, stress management, and improved sleep quality can help women navigate this challenging period. By adopting a proactive approach to weight management, women can enhance their overall health and quality of life during menopause and beyond, embodying elegance and resilience through every stage.

Skin and Hair Changes

During menopause, many women face transformative changes in their skin and hair, which can be unsettling and impact their self-esteem. These shifts are predominantly driven by hormonal fluctuations, particularly the decline in estrogen levels, which are essential for maintaining skin and hair vitality.

One of the most prominent skin changes during menopause is increased dryness. Estrogen plays a pivotal role in retaining the skin's moisture by promoting natural oil production and enhancing the skin's ability to hold water. As estrogen levels wane, the skin loses moisture more rapidly, resulting in dryness, roughness, and a dull complexion. This exacerbates the appearance of fine lines and wrinkles, contributing to an aged look. Additionally, the skin's natural barrier function weakens, making it more vulnerable to irritants and environmental damage.

Another significant transformation is the reduction in collagen and elastin production. Collagen provides structural integrity to the skin, while elastin allows it to remain supple and resilient. With lower estrogen levels, the synthesis of these proteins diminishes, leading to a loss of firmness and elasticity. The skin becomes thinner and more prone to sagging, particularly in areas like the cheeks, jawline, and neck, resulting in deeper wrinkles and more pronounced fine lines.

Hyperpigmentation or age spots are also prevalent during menopause. Estrogen regulates melanin production, the pigment responsible for skin color. When estrogen levels decline, melanin production can become uneven, causing dark spots and an overall uneven skin tone. These age spots are especially noticeable on areas frequently exposed to the sun, such as the face, hands, and arms.

Hair changes during menopause can be equally disconcerting. Many women experience hair thinning or hair loss, attributable to the decrease in estrogen and the relative increase in androgens, or male hormones. These hormonal shifts can lead to androgenic alopecia, where hair follicles shrink and produce finer, shorter strands. This results in noticeable thinning on the scalp, particularly at the crown and along the part line. Additionally, the hair growth cycle can become disrupted, with more hair in the resting phase and less in the active growing phase, leading to increased shedding.

Menopause also affects hair texture and quality. Reduced estrogen levels decrease sebum production, the natural oil that keeps hair hydrated and shiny. Consequently, hair may become drier, more brittle, and prone to breakage. Some women may notice changes in their hair's texture, such as increased coarseness or a loss of natural curl or wave.

To manage these skin and hair changes, adopting a targeted skincare and haircare routine is essential. For the skin, using products focused on hydration and barrier repair can alleviate dryness and improve texture. Ingredients like hyaluronic acid, glycerin, and ceramides enhance moisture retention and support the skin's natural barrier. Incorporating retinoids or peptides stimulates collagen production and improves skin firmness. Regular use of broad-spectrum sunscreen is crucial to prevent further hyperpigmentation and protect against UV damage.

For hair care, gentle cleansing and conditioning products designed to add moisture and strengthen hair can mitigate dryness and breakage. Avoiding harsh treatments like excessive heat styling and chemical processing protects hair health. Incorporating scalp massages and using products with ingredients like minoxidil or natural oils may promote hair growth and improve overall hair density.

The skin and hair changes experienced during menopause are primarily driven by hormonal fluctuations, leading to increased dryness, loss of elasticity, hyperpigmentation, and hair thinning. By understanding these changes and adopting appropriate skincare and haircare routines, women can manage these effects and maintain their appearance and confidence during this transitional phase of life.

Emotional and Mental Health

Mood Swings and Anxiety

Menopause marks a pivotal transition in a woman's life, often bringing a cascade of physical and emotional changes. Among the most challenging of these are mood swings and anxiety, which can profoundly impact daily life and overall well-being. These emotional disturbances stem primarily from hormonal fluctuations, particularly the decline in estrogen and progesterone levels.

Estrogen plays a vital role in mood regulation by influencing the production and activity of neurotransmitters such as serotonin, dopamine, and norepinephrine. These neurotransmitters are essential for maintaining emotional stability and a sense of well-being. As estrogen levels drop during menopause, the production and regulation of these neurotransmitters can become erratic, leading to mood swings. Women may find themselves feeling irritable, sad, or angry for no apparent reason, and these mood changes can occur suddenly and unpredictably. This emotional volatility can strain personal relationships, hinder concentration at work, and diminish overall quality of life.

Anxiety is another prevalent emotional symptom during menopause. The hormonal shifts that occur can trigger feelings of nervousness, worry, and fear. Some women may experience generalized anxiety, where they feel anxious about various aspects of life without a specific trigger. Others might suffer from panic attacks, characterized by sudden, intense episodes of fear accompanied by physical symptoms such as heart palpitations, shortness of breath, and dizziness. These anxiety symptoms can be debilitating, making it difficult to engage in everyday activities and increasing the risk of developing other mental health issues such as depression.

Sleep disturbances, which are also common during menopause, can exacerbate mood swings and anxiety. Hot flashes and night sweats can interrupt sleep, leading to insomnia or poor-quality rest. Chronic sleep deprivation can significantly affect mood, making women more prone to irritability and anxiety. The lack of restorative sleep can also impair cognitive function, leading to difficulties with memory, concentration, and decision-making, further contributing to emotional distress.

The psychosocial impact of menopause can also contribute to mood swings and anxiety. For many women, menopause signifies the end of their reproductive years, which can evoke feelings of loss and a sense of aging. This transition can lead to reflections on life changes, body image concerns, and fears about health and mortality. The societal stigma surrounding menopause and aging can also make women feel isolated and unsupported during this time, further heightening feelings of anxiety and mood instability.

Managing mood swings and anxiety during menopause often requires a multifaceted approach. Lifestyle modifications, such as regular physical activity, can help stabilize mood and reduce anxiety. Exercise promotes the release of endorphins, which are natural mood elevators, and helps reduce stress. A balanced diet rich in nutrients that support brain health, such as omega-3 fatty acids, can also be beneficial. Practicing mindfulness and relaxation techniques, such as yoga, meditation, and deep breathing exercises, can help manage stress and improve emotional resilience.

Therapy and counseling can provide valuable support for women experiencing severe mood swings and anxiety during menopause. Cognitive-behavioral therapy (CBT) is particularly effective in helping women develop coping strategies and change negative thought patterns. For some women, medication may be necessary. Hormone replacement therapy (HRT) can help alleviate severe mood swings and anxiety by stabilizing hormone levels, although it is not suitable for everyone and should be discussed with a healthcare provider. Antidepressants and anti-anxiety medications may also be prescribed to help manage symptoms.

Mood swings and anxiety are common but challenging aspects of menopause, driven by hormonal changes and psychosocial factors. Understanding the underlying causes and adopting a comprehensive approach to managing these symptoms can help women navigate this transitional period more smoothly and maintain their emotional well-being. With the right support and strategies, it is possible to mitigate the impact of mood swings and anxiety, allowing women to lead fulfilling lives during and after menopause.

Memory and Cognitive Function

Menopause, a transformative period in a woman's life, is often accompanied by not only physical changes but also notable shifts in cognitive function. Many women find themselves grappling with memory lapses, difficulties in concentration, and a pervasive sense of cognitive decline during this phase. These alterations can be distressing, impacting daily life significantly. Therefore, understanding the root causes and exploring effective management strategies is essential for navigating this transition with grace.

The decline in estrogen levels is a primary factor behind the cognitive changes during menopause. Estrogen is integral to brain function, influencing memory, attention, and executive processes. It has a profound impact on the hippocampus, a brain region crucial for memory formation and retrieval. As estrogen levels wane, the efficiency of these cognitive processes diminishes, leading to noticeable memory and cognitive performance changes.

Memory issues during menopause often manifest as frequent forgetfulness or difficulty recalling names and words. Many women find themselves misplacing items, missing appointments, or struggling to remember recent conversations' details. This phenomenon, often termed "brain fog," can be particularly frustrating, affecting confidence and productivity in both personal and professional realms. Multitasking and focusing on complex tasks also become more challenging, exacerbating feelings of cognitive decline.

Stress and sleep disturbances, common during menopause, further contribute to cognitive issues. Chronic stress impairs cognitive function by affecting the prefrontal cortex, the brain region responsible for decision-making, planning, and social behavior regulation. Sleep disturbances, including insomnia and frequent awakenings due to night sweats, lead to sleep deprivation. Poor sleep quality negatively impacts cognitive processes such as attention, problem-solving, and memory consolidation, making it difficult to think clearly and retain information.

Moreover, the psychosocial changes accompanying menopause, such as anxiety and depression, amplify cognitive difficulties. Emotional stress can hinder concentration and information processing. Additionally, changes in self-perception and body image during menopause can add to the psychological burden, potentially leading to decreased cognitive performance.

Despite these challenges, several strategies can mitigate the impact of menopause on memory and cognitive function. Regular physical exercise is one of the most effective ways to support brain health. Exercise boosts blood flow to the brain, promotes the growth of new neurons, and enhances neuronal connectivity, improving memory, attention, and overall cognitive function.

A healthy diet is equally crucial. Consuming foods rich in antioxidants, omega-3 fatty acids, and other brain-supporting nutrients can help preserve cognitive function. Incorporating fish, nuts, seeds, fruits, and vegetables into your diet is particularly beneficial. Additionally, staying mentally active through reading, puzzles, and learning new skills keeps the brain engaged and promotes cognitive resilience.

Stress management techniques such as mindfulness, meditation, and yoga are vital for maintaining cognitive function. These practices reduce stress levels and improve emotional well-being, enhancing cognitive performance. Ensuring adequate sleep is also essential; establishing good sleep hygiene can significantly improve sleep quality.

For some women, hormone replacement therapy (HRT) may alleviate severe cognitive symptoms. HRT can help stabilize hormone levels and potentially improve cognitive function, although it is not suitable for everyone and should be considered carefully with a healthcare provider.

In essence, menopause can bring significant changes in memory and cognitive function due to hormonal fluctuations, stress, and sleep disturbances. By understanding these changes and adopting a holistic approach that includes physical exercise, a healthy diet, stress management, and possibly medical interventions, women can maintain cognitive health during this transitional period. Addressing these cognitive challenges proactively enables women to lead active, fulfilling lives throughout menopause and beyond.

Depression and Emotional Well-being

Depression and emotional well-being are paramount during the menopause transition, a phase that demands our full attention and care. Menopause, the natural biological milestone signaling the end of a woman's reproductive years, ushers in profound hormonal shifts that can significantly influence mental health. The drop-in estrogen levels is particularly impactful, given estrogen's critical role in maintaining mood and emotional balance.

During menopause, many women encounter mood swings, irritability, and an overarching sense of emotional turbulence. These fluctuations can span from mild moodiness to severe depression, disrupting daily life and diminishing quality of life. The hormonal changes can lead to a decline in serotonin levels, the neurotransmitter essential for mood regulation. Reduced serotonin often results in feelings of sadness, anxiety, and depression.

Depression during menopause manifests in diverse ways. Some women might experience persistent sadness or hopelessness, while others might lose interest in activities that once brought joy. Common symptoms also include fatigue, difficulty concentrating, appetite changes, and sleep disturbances. These emotional hurdles are often intertwined with physical symptoms like hot flashes, night sweats, and vaginal dryness, which further disrupt sleep and daily routines, creating a relentless cycle of discomfort.

The emotional turmoil of menopause isn't solely biological. This transition often coincides with pivotal life events, such as children leaving the nest, caring for aging parents, and shifts in career or personal relationships. These stressors can amplify feelings of depression and anxiety. Moreover, societal perceptions of aging and menopause can foster a sense of loss and diminished self-worth, further undermining emotional well-being.

Addressing depression and emotional well-being during menopause necessitates a holistic approach. Open dialogue with healthcare providers is crucial. Women should feel empowered to discuss their emotional and psychological symptoms as candidly as their physical ones. Mental health professionals can provide indispensable support through counseling, cognitive-behavioral therapy, or medication when needed. Antidepressants or other medications may be prescribed to manage severe symptoms of depression and anxiety.

Lifestyle changes play a vital role in enhancing emotional well-being. Regular physical exercise is a potent antidote to depression. Exercise triggers the release of endorphins, the body's natural mood elevators, which counteract the effects of declining estrogen. Additionally, physical activity improves sleep quality, reduces stress, and boosts self-esteem.

A nutritious diet rich in brain-supporting nutrients is equally important. Foods high in omega-3 fatty acids, such as fish and flaxseeds, have mood-stabilizing benefits. Incorporating a variety of fruits, vegetables, whole grains, and lean proteins ensures the body receives essential nutrients for overall health and emotional stability.

Stress management techniques like mindfulness meditation, yoga, and deep-breathing exercises can also mitigate symptoms of depression and anxiety. These practices foster relaxation and emotional equilibrium, helping women navigate menopause's emotional ebb and flow. Social support is another crucial element. Connecting with friends, family, or support groups fosters a sense of community and understanding, alleviating feelings of isolation.

Depression and emotional well-being during menopause are influenced by both hormonal shifts and life changes. A comprehensive strategy encompassing medical support, lifestyle adjustments, stress management, and social connections is essential for managing these emotional challenges. By addressing both the physical and emotional dimensions of menopause, women can navigate this transition with greater resilience and well-being, maintaining a positive outlook on their mental health and overall quality of life.

CHAPTER 3

Managing Menopausal Symptoms

Hormone Replacement Therapy (HRT)

Benefits and Risks

When considering any health intervention, it is paramount to balance both the benefits and the risks to make an informed decision. This principle is especially pertinent for menopause management, where options span from hormone replacement therapy (HRT) to lifestyle modifications, alternative treatments, and more. Gaining a comprehensive understanding of the advantages and potential drawbacks of these treatments can empower women to navigate this life transition with confidence and elegance.

Hormone replacement therapy remains one of the most prevalent treatments for alleviating menopause symptoms. HRT involves administering estrogen, or a combination of estrogen and progesterone, to mitigate symptoms such as hot flashes, night sweats, and vaginal dryness. The primary allure of HRT lies in its effectiveness; it significantly alleviates these distressing symptoms, thereby enhancing the quality of life for many women. Moreover, HRT can help prevent bone loss, reducing the risk of osteoporosis and fractures, common concerns in the post-menopausal phase.

However, HRT is not without its shadows. Studies have indicated that HRT can elevate the risk of certain conditions, including breast cancer, heart disease, stroke, and blood clots. The risk profile is nuanced and varies depending on factors such as the type of hormones used, the duration of therapy, and the individual's health history. For instance, women who initiate HRT closer to the onset of menopause may face different risk levels compared to those who start later. Hence, it is crucial for women to have in-depth discussions with their healthcare providers to assess their personal risk factors and determine whether HRT is a suitable option.

Beyond HRT, lifestyle changes offer a more natural approach to managing menopause symptoms, with their own set of benefits and minimal risks. Regular physical exercise can aid in weight management, enhance mood, and strengthen bones, thereby countering some adverse effects of menopause. A balanced diet rich in calcium, vitamin D, and other nutrients supports overall health and helps maintain bone density. The benefits of these lifestyle adjustments extend well beyond menopause, fostering long-term health and vitality.

While the risks associated with lifestyle changes are generally minimal, their consistent implementation can be challenging. For instance, maintaining a regular exercise routine or making significant dietary changes demands commitment and motivation, which can be particularly taxing during periods of low energy or depression, both common during menopause.

Alternative treatments, such as herbal supplements and acupuncture, have garnered popularity among women seeking natural relief from menopause symptoms. Herbal remedies like black cohosh and red clover are reputed to alleviate hot flashes and mood swings, while acupuncture is reported to assist with a range of symptoms, including hot flashes and insomnia. The allure of these alternative treatments lies in their natural origins and the perception of being safer than pharmaceuticals.

Nevertheless, the risks of alternative treatments should not be underestimated. The efficacy and safety of many herbal supplements are not well-documented, and some may interact with medications or cause side effects. Acupuncture, although generally safe when performed by a qualified practitioner, can lead to complications if improperly done. It is crucial for women to consult with healthcare providers before embarking on any alternative treatment to ensure it is safe and appropriate for their individual health needs.

The benefits and risks of menopause treatments are diverse and influenced by individual health profiles and preferences. HRT can provide substantial symptom relief but comes with significant risks that need careful consideration. Lifestyle changes promote overall health and well-being with minimal risks, though they require dedication and effort. Alternative treatments offer natural options but need thorough evaluation for safety and efficacy. By understanding the full spectrum of benefits and risks, women can make informed decisions that best support their health and quality of life during menopause, navigating this transition with grace and poise.

Different Types of HRT

Hormone Replacement Therapy (HRT) is the pinnacle of modern treatment, crafted to alleviate the myriad symptoms of menopause by restoring the body's diminishing levels of hormones, primarily estrogen and progesterone. For the discerning woman exploring this sophisticated therapy, understanding the diverse types of HRT is essential. The choice of treatment not only influences its efficacy but also the potential risks involved.

A key distinction in HRT lies between systemic and local treatments. Systemic HRT involves hormones that circulate through the bloodstream, reaching various organs and tissues. This approach is typically employed to address a broad spectrum of menopausal symptoms, such as hot flashes, night sweats, mood swings, and osteoporosis. Systemic HRT can be administered in multiple forms, including oral tablets, transdermal patches, gels, and injections. Each method boasts its own set of advantages. Oral tablets offer convenience but may increase the risk of liver-related side effects. Conversely, transdermal patches provide a steady release of hormones and are less likely to impact liver function, making them a preferred option for many women.

Local HRT, on the other hand, targets specific areas of the body, particularly the vaginal region, to treat localized symptoms such as vaginal dryness, itching, and discomfort during intercourse. This therapy is usually delivered via creams, rings, or tablets applied or inserted directly into the vagina. Given that local HRT delivers hormones in low doses directly to the site of symptoms, it typically has fewer systemic effects and is often considered safer for women experiencing primarily genitourinary symptoms.

Another pivotal distinction in HRT is between estrogen-only therapy and combined estrogen-progesterone therapy. Estrogen-only HRT is generally prescribed for women who have undergone a hysterectomy, thereby eliminating the risk of developing endometrial cancer, heightened by estrogen use without progesterone. This therapy can effectively alleviate many menopausal symptoms and aid in preventing bone loss. For women with an intact uterus, however, combined HRT—which includes both estrogen and progesterone—is recommended to mitigate the increased risk of endometrial cancer associated with estrogen-only therapy. The addition of progesterone helps protect the endometrial lining by countering the proliferative effects of estrogen.

Within combined HRT, there are further nuances, including sequential and continuous combined regimens. Sequential combined HRT involves taking estrogen continuously and adding progesterone for part of the cycle, typically for 12-14 days each month, often resulting in a regular monthly bleed similar to a menstrual period. Continuous combined HRT, on the other hand, entails taking both estrogen and progesterone every day without interruption, usually leading to the absence of bleeding after an initial adjustment period. The choice between these regimens depends on the woman's symptoms, medical history, and preference regarding bleeding patterns.

There is also the allure of bioidentical hormones, which are chemically identical to those produced by the human body. These can be synthesized from plant sources and are available in both standard pharmaceutical preparations and custom-compounded forms. Some women favor bioidentical hormones, believing them to be more natural and potentially less risky, though there is ongoing debate and research regarding their safety and efficacy compared to conventional HRT.

The decision to embark on HRT and the selection of a specific therapy type should be made in close collaboration with a healthcare provider, considering the individual's symptoms, health risks, and personal preferences. Regular follow-up is crucial to monitor the therapy's effectiveness and adjust the treatment as necessary to ensure optimal outcomes and minimize potential risks. By understanding the various types of HRT, women can make informed decisions, managing their menopause symptoms with confidence and sophistication.

Finding the Right Dosage and Monitoring

Finding the right dosage of Hormone Replacement Therapy (HRT) and ensuring meticulous monitoring are quintessential aspects of managing menopause symptoms with finesse. This process demands a personalized approach, as each woman's journey through menopause is distinct, and their response to HRT can vary dramatically. The objective is to attain symptom relief while minimizing potential risks, necessitating a delicate balance and continuous evaluation.

When embarking on HRT, healthcare providers generally commence with the lowest effective dose. This cautious approach helps minimize potential side effects and allows the body to acclimate to the hormone supplementation. The initial dosage is often determined by the severity of the woman's symptoms, her overall health, and her medical history. For example, women with milder symptoms might start with a lower dose, whereas those experiencing more severe symptoms might require a slightly higher starting point. The selection of hormone types and delivery methods—be it oral, transdermal, or local—also influences the initial dosing strategy.

Once HRT is initiated, vigilant monitoring is paramount to assess its efficacy and safety. Follow-up appointments are usually scheduled within the first few months to evaluate how well the therapy is working and to detect any adverse effects. During these consultations, the healthcare provider will discuss the patient's symptom relief, any side effects encountered, and overall well-being. It is imperative for women to communicate openly about their symptoms and any changes they notice, as this feedback is crucial for making necessary adjustments to the therapy.

Finding the optimal dosage often involves a series of adjustments. If symptoms persist or side effects become problematic, the dosage may be modified. This could entail increasing the dose to enhance symptom control or decreasing it to alleviate side effects. In certain instances, changing the type of hormones or the delivery method might be required. For example, a woman experiencing gastrointestinal side effects from oral HRT might find better results with a transdermal patch, which bypasses the digestive system.

Hormone levels can also be monitored through blood tests, though this is not always standard practice. These tests measure the concentrations of estrogen and progesterone in the bloodstream, providing objective data that can assist in fine-tuning the therapy. However, the alleviation of symptoms and overall health improvements are often more critical indicators of the appropriate dosage than hormone levels alone.

In addition to monitoring hormone levels, regular health screenings are essential for women on HRT. These include mammograms, pelvic exams, and bone density assessments, as prolonged HRT can influence the risk profiles for conditions such as breast cancer and osteoporosis. Blood pressure and cholesterol levels should also be monitored regularly, given the potential cardiovascular implications of hormone therapy.

The importance of a tailored approach cannot be overstated. Factors such as age, body mass index, coexisting medical conditions, and lifestyle habits all influence how a woman metabolizes hormones. For instance, smoking can affect estrogen metabolism, necessitating dosage adjustments. Similarly, changes in weight or the onset of new medical conditions might require modifications to the therapy.

Women should be encouraged to maintain a healthy lifestyle to complement their HRT. Regular physical activity, a balanced diet rich in calcium and vitamin D, smoking cessation, and limiting alcohol intake can enhance the benefits of hormone therapy and contribute to overall health.

Ultimately, finding the right dosage of HRT is a dynamic process that evolves over time. Consistent communication between the woman and her healthcare provider is essential to navigate this journey successfully. By carefully adjusting dosages and closely monitoring health outcomes, women can achieve effective symptom relief and enhance their quality of life during and after the menopausal transition.

Non-Hormonal Treatments

Natural Remedies and Supplements

Natural remedies and supplements offer an elegant and holistic approach to managing menopause symptoms, providing a chic alternative or complement to hormone replacement therapy (HRT). For many discerning women, the allure of these natural options lies in their potential to mitigate concerns associated with synthetic hormones. Delving into natural remedies can deliver not only symptom relief but also bolster overall well-being during the menopausal transition.

Herbal supplements are at the forefront of natural menopause solutions, each offering unique benefits that seamlessly integrate into a sophisticated wellness routine. Black cohosh is a perennial favorite, celebrated for its potential to ease hot flashes and night sweats. Esteemed for its estrogen-mimicking properties, this herb offers a naturally graceful solution to common menopausal discomforts. Red clover, another chic choice, brims with phytoestrogens—plant compounds that echo the effects of estrogen. This vibrant supplement is known to alleviate hot flashes and may even contribute to enhanced bone health. Meanwhile, evening primrose oil, rich in gamma-linolenic acid, is a promising contender for alleviating mood swings and breast tenderness, though further research is warranted to fully unveil its benefits.

Soy, with its versatile and stylish appeal, stands out as a dietary gem in the realm of natural menopause remedies. Isoflavones, the phytoestrogens found in soy products like tofu, soy milk, and edamame, are believed to harmonize hormone levels and diminish hot flashes. Flaxseed, another nutritional powerhouse, is abundant in lignans—phytoestrogens that can be seamlessly incorporated into the diet to support hormonal balance and manage menopausal symptoms with grace.

Embracing a balanced diet rich in essential vitamins and minerals can have a transformative impact on menopause symptoms. Calcium and vitamin D are indispensable for maintaining bone health, an increasing priority as estrogen levels wane and osteoporosis risk rises. Magnesium, present in leafy greens, nuts, and seeds, can alleviate sleep disturbances and muscle cramps. Vitamin E, with its potent antioxidant properties, may reduce the severity of hot flashes and night sweats, adding a touch of luminosity to one's wellness regimen.

Lifestyle modifications are the cornerstone of natural menopause management, enhancing both physical and emotional well-being. Regular physical activity—whether it's an invigorating walk, a refreshing swim, or a serene yoga session—helps maintain a healthy weight, uplift mood, and elevate overall wellness. Exercise has been shown to reduce the frequency and intensity of hot flashes and improve sleep quality. Stress management techniques such as mindfulness, meditation, and deep breathing exercises offer a sophisticated means to alleviate anxiety and mood swings commonly associated with menopause.

Acupuncture, a revered practice in traditional Chinese medicine, is another natural remedy embraced by many women. This ancient art involves the delicate insertion of thin needles into specific points on the body to balance energy flow. Emerging studies suggest that acupuncture can reduce hot flashes, enhance sleep, and alleviate mood disturbances, possibly by stimulating the release of endorphins and fostering relaxation.

For women considering natural remedies and supplements, a consultation with a healthcare provider is indispensable. Despite their natural origins, these remedies can have side effects and may interact with other medications. A healthcare provider can offer personalized guidance, ensuring that the chosen remedies are both safe and effective.

Natural remedies and supplements offer an elegant and effective approach to managing menopause symptoms. By incorporating herbal supplements, thoughtful dietary changes, and holistic lifestyle modifications, women can navigate menopause with poise and confidence. However, it is essential to approach these remedies with a discerning eye and under professional guidance to ensure their safety and efficacy. With a well-rounded, sophisticated approach that blends natural and medical strategies, women can embrace the challenges of menopause with grace and assurance.

Diet and Nutrition for Symptom Relief

Diet and nutrition are the cornerstones of managing and alleviating menopause symptoms with sophistication and grace. As women navigate through menopause, their bodies undergo significant hormonal shifts, leading to a myriad of symptoms such as hot flashes, weight gain, mood swings, and bone density loss. By making intentional and stylish dietary choices, women can support their bodies through these changes and enhance their overall well-being.

One of the most notorious symptoms of menopause is the hot flash, which can strike with both frequency and intensity. Certain foods and beverages can exacerbate these fiery episodes. Caffeine, alcohol, and spicy foods are well-known triggers, and reducing or eliminating these items from one's diet can help decrease the frequency and severity of hot flashes. Instead, a chic and nutritious diet rich in fruits, vegetables, whole grains, and lean proteins can provide essential nutrients that support hormonal balance and overall vitality.

Phytoestrogens, those elegant plant compounds that mimic estrogen's actions in the body, are a woman's best friend during menopause. Incorporating foods high in phytoestrogens can offer relief from menopausal symptoms. Soy products like tofu, soy milk, and edamame are fabulous sources of phytoestrogens and can help ease hot flashes and night sweats. Flaxseeds are another excellent source, and their subtle, nutty flavor can easily be added to smoothies, cereals, or yogurt. Including these foods in the diet may help mitigate some of the discomforts associated with decreased estrogen levels.

Maintaining a healthy weight becomes increasingly paramount during menopause, as hormonal changes can lead to weight gain, particularly around the abdomen. A diet high in fiber can aid in weight management by promoting satiety and reducing overall calorie intake. Whole grains, legumes, fruits, and vegetables are not only high in dietary fiber but also bursting with vitamins, minerals, and antioxidants that support overall health and a radiant appearance.

Calcium and vitamin D are essential nutrients for preserving bone health, a critical concern during menopause due to the heightened risk of osteoporosis. As estrogen levels wane, bone density can decrease, making bones more susceptible to fractures. Dairy products like milk, yogurt, and cheese are classic sources of calcium. For those who are lactose intolerant or prefer non-dairy options, fortified plant-based milks, leafy green vegetables, and almonds are also rich in calcium. Vitamin D, the sunshine vitamin, can be absorbed from sunlight, but dietary sources such as fatty fish, egg yolks, and fortified foods are also crucial. Adequate calcium and vitamin D intake can help maintain bone density and reduce the risk of osteoporosis.

Omega-3 fatty acids, the stylish anti-inflammatory agents found in fatty fish like salmon, mackerel, and sardines, as well as in walnuts and flaxseeds, can help improve mood and cognitive function. These healthy fats also support heart health, which becomes increasingly important as cardiovascular risk rises post-menopause. Including these foods in the diet can provide both physical and mental health benefits, enhancing one's sense of well-being and elegance.

Hydration is another vital aspect of diet and nutrition during menopause. Drinking plenty of water can help manage hot flashes and maintain overall hydration. Hydration is also beneficial for skin health, which can be affected by hormonal changes, leading to dryness and loss of elasticity. Sipping on chic, refreshing water infused with cucumber or lemon can add a touch of glamour to staying hydrated.

Lastly, reducing sugar and refined carbohydrates can help manage blood sugar levels and reduce the risk of insulin resistance, which can become more prevalent during menopause. Opting for complex carbohydrates like whole grains and limiting the intake of sugary snacks and beverages can support metabolic health and prevent energy fluctuations, ensuring you feel your best throughout the day.

Diet and nutrition are powerful allies in the journey through menopause. By making informed and stylish dietary choices, women can support their bodies through this transition and elevate their quality of life. A balanced diet rich in phytoestrogens, fiber, calcium, vitamin D, omega-3 fatty acids, and adequate hydration can alleviate many menopause symptoms and promote overall health and well-being, allowing women to navigate this phase with confidence and grace.

Exercise and Physical Activity

Exercise and physical activity are the chic cornerstones of a radiant, healthy lifestyle, especially during the transformative journey of menopause. As women gracefully transition through this life phase, regular physical activity emerges as a glamorous remedy, alleviating myriad menopausal symptoms, enhancing overall well-being, and slashing the risk of chronic diseases with elegance and style.

One of the most alluring benefits of exercise during menopause is its sleek ability to help manage weight. Hormonal changes often usher in unwanted weight gain, particularly around the abdomen, increasing the risk of cardiovascular disease and diabetes. Regular physical activity works like couture tailoring for your body, regulating weight by boosting metabolism and promoting calorie burn. Aerobic exercises such as walking, jogging, cycling, and swimming are the haute couture of fitness, particularly effective in maintaining a svelte figure. These activities not only torch calories but also elevate cardiovascular health by strengthening the heart and enhancing circulation.

But let's not forget the allure of strength training. As estrogen levels wane, the risk of losing muscle mass and bone density surges, paving the way for conditions like osteoporosis. Strength training exercises—think weight lifting, resistance band workouts, and bodyweight exercises like push-ups and squats—are the must-have accessories in a menopausal woman's fitness wardrobe. These exercises stimulate the growth of new bone tissue, sculpting muscles and fortifying bones, preventing fractures, and maintaining mobility and independence as women age gracefully.

Flexibility and balance exercises add the final touch of finesse to a well-rounded fitness routine. Yoga, Pilates, and tai chi are the little black dresses of exercise—timeless and essential. They not only enhance flexibility and balance but also elevate mental well-being. Yoga, in particular, is a serene sanctuary for the mind, reducing stress, anxiety, and depression, which can be frequent companions during menopause. The mindful breathing and meditative aspects of yoga calm the mind and uplift the spirit, making joint pain and stiffness—common due to hormonal changes and aging—fade into the background.

The impact of exercise on sleep quality is nothing short of transformative. Menopause often brings disruptive symptoms like night sweats and insomnia, turning beauty sleep into a rare commodity. Regular physical activity regulates the sleep-wake cycle, making it easier to drift into a deep, restorative slumber. It also diminishes the severity of night sweats and hot flashes, ensuring better rest. Engaging in moderate-intensity exercise during the day can lead to a night of beauty sleep that rivals the rejuvenation of the most luxurious spa treatments.

The mental health benefits of exercise during menopause are simply sublime. Women may experience mood swings, anxiety, and depression during this phase, but physical activity serves as a natural elixir. Exercise triggers the release of endorphins, those fabulous "feel-good" hormones that elevate mood and reduce pain perception. It also boosts serotonin and dopamine levels, the chic neurotransmitters that regulate mood and create a sense of well-being.

Finding an exercise routine that feels as fabulous as a designer dress is essential for long-term commitment. Consistency is the key to unlocking the full benefits of physical activity. Aim to blend a variety of exercises into your routine, addressing cardiovascular fitness, strength, flexibility, and balance. Consulting with a healthcare provider or a fitness professional can help tailor a bespoke exercise plan that complements your health status, fitness levels, and personal preferences.

Excrcise and physical activity are the quintessential elements of managing menopause symptoms and promoting overall health. By embracing an active lifestyle, women can enhance their physical fitness, elevate their mental well-being, and reduce the risk of chronic diseases with the grace and poise of a runway model. A balanced exercise routine that includes aerobic, strengt   ah, flexibility, and balance exercises will help women navigate the challenges of menopause with unparalleled ease, maintaining a high quality of life with flair.

Alternative and Complementary Therapies

Acupuncture and Herbal Medicine

Acupuncture and herbal medicine, cherished pillars of traditional Chinese medicine, have been the go-to solutions for a myriad of health issues, including the ever-challenging menopausal symptoms. These elegant, natural therapies serve as either a chic alternative or a sophisticated complement to conventional treatments, offering holistic relief with a touch of ancient wisdom.

Acupuncture, the artful practice of inserting fine needles into precise points on the body, aims to stimulate energy flow and restore inner harmony. This time-honored technique is rooted in the concept of Qi (pronounced "chee"), the life force that courses through the body's meridians or pathways. In traditional Chinese medicine, menopause is viewed as a disruption in the delicate balance of Yin and Yang, the elemental forces governing bodily functions. By meticulously targeting specific acupuncture points, practitioners strive to harmonize these energies, mitigate symptoms, and elevate overall health.

For menopausal women, one of acupuncture's most celebrated benefits is its prowess in quelling hot flashes and night sweats. These bothersome symptoms, hallmark challenges of menopause, can significantly impair quality of life. Research has illuminated that acupuncture can diminish the frequency and intensity of hot flashes by recalibrating the body's temperature control mechanisms and modulating hormonal activity. Furthermore, acupuncture's prowess extends to enhancing sleep quality, often compromised by night sweats and insomnia. By fostering relaxation and diminishing stress, acupuncture aids menopausal women in achieving restful and rejuvenating sleep.

Acupuncture also excels in alleviating mood swings, anxiety, and depression, which frequently accompany menopause due to hormonal upheavals. The practice prompts the release of endorphins and serotonin, neurotransmitters that uplift mood and engender a sense of well-being. This natural elevation of feel-good chemicals can stabilize mood and alleviate the emotional turbulence that many women face during menopause.

Herbal medicine, another cornerstone of traditional Chinese medicine, offers substantial benefits for menopausal women. These remedies are meticulously tailored to individual needs following a comprehensive assessment by a trained practitioner. Noteworthy herbs include black cohosh, red clover, dong quai, and ginseng, each with unique properties targeting specific symptoms.

Black cohosh is renowned for its efficacy in reducing hot flashes and night sweats, thanks to its phytoestrogens plant-based compounds mimicking estrogen's effects in the body. Red clover, also rich in phytoestrogens, helps alleviate hot flashes, improve bone density, and bolster cardiovascular health. Dong quai, often dubbed the "female ginseng," is prized for regulating menstrual cycles and relieving symptoms like hot flashes and vaginal dryness. Ginseng itself is celebrated for boosting energy, reducing fatigue, and enhancing overall vitality, including cognitive function, which may wane during menopause due to hormonal shifts.

Herbal medicine practitioners often blend these potent herbs into bespoke formulas, meticulously designed to address each woman's unique symptoms and health profile. The synergistic combination of acupuncture and herbal medicine offers a comprehensive approach to managing menopause. While acupuncture fine-tunes the body's energy pathways and internal equilibrium, herbal medicine delivers targeted relief through the potent properties of plants, collectively fostering overall health and well-being.

It's paramount to seek these therapies from qualified practitioners. Accurate diagnosis and tailored treatment plans are essential to ensure safety and efficacy. Women intrigued by these sophisticated remedies should consult licensed acupuncturists and herbalists with a proven track record in treating menopausal symptoms.

In essence, acupuncture and herbal medicine stand as invaluable options for women desiring natural remedies for menopause. By addressing the root causes of symptoms and promoting holistic balance, these therapies can significantly enhance quality of life during the menopausal transition. With the guidance of skilled practitioners, women can harness the benefits of these ancient practices, navigating menopause with grace, ease, and well-being.

Mindfulness, Meditation and Yoga

Mindfulness, meditation, and yoga have emerged as the ultimate trifecta for managing the physical and emotional challenges of menopause. These ancient practices offer holistic, sophisticated approaches to health that cater to both mind and body. For women navigating the turbulent waters of menopause, these techniques can provide substantial relief and elevate overall well-being.

Mindfulness is all about being fully present in the moment, tuning into your thoughts, feelings, and sensations without judgment. During menopause—a time often marked by hormonal fluctuations and emotional upheaval—mindfulness can be a game-changer. By cultivating mindfulness, women can gain greater control over their reactions to stress and anxiety. This practice can be especially beneficial for managing mood swings and irritability, common symptoms during menopause. Regular mindfulness sessions can also enhance sleep quality, which is frequently disrupted during this life stage.

Meditation, closely intertwined with mindfulness, involves focused attention and relaxation techniques that help to calm the mind. Through meditation, women can significantly reduce stress and anxiety, lower blood pressure, and cultivate a deep sense of peace and well-being. Various forms of meditation, such as guided visualization, loving-kindness meditation, and body scan meditation, each offer unique benefits. For menopausal women, a daily meditation practice can serve as a sanctuary from the pressures of daily life and a means to reconnect with their inner selves. The advantages of meditation extend beyond emotional balance; it can also enhance cognitive function, a particularly valuable benefit as some women experience memory lapses and concentration difficulties during menopause.

Yoga elegantly combines physical postures, breath control, and meditation to promote overall health and well-being. It offers a comprehensive approach to managing menopausal symptoms. The physical aspect of yoga helps maintain flexibility, strength, and balance, which can decline with age and hormonal changes. Specific yoga poses can alleviate common menopausal discomforts such as hot flashes, joint pain, and stiffness. For instance, restorative poses and forward bends are known to have a cooling effect on the body, providing relief from hot flashes. Inversions and supported poses can help with sleep disturbances by promoting relaxation and reducing stress.

Beyond the physical benefits, yoga's focus on breath work and meditation can significantly impact emotional health. Pranayama, or breath control, is a fundamental aspect of yoga that can help regulate the nervous system and reduce stress. Techniques like alternate nostril breathing and deep belly breathing can be particularly calming, helping to manage anxiety and mood swings. The meditative aspect of yoga fosters a sense of inner peace and self-awareness, which can be empowering during the menopausal transition.

Engaging in mindfulness, meditation, and yoga can also foster a sense of community and support. Many women find solace in attending yoga classes or meditation groups, where they can share their experiences and learn from others going through similar life stages. This sense of connection can alleviate feelings of isolation and provide a valuable support network.

Incorporating these practices into daily life does not require a significant time commitment. Even a few minutes of mindfulness or meditation each day can make a substantial difference.

For yoga, short, regular sessions can be just as beneficial as longer, less frequent practice. The key is consistency and finding what works best for the individual.

Mindfulness, meditation and yoga offer powerful, natural methods for managing the myriad symptoms of menopause. These practices not only address physical discomforts but also promote emotional resilience and mental clarity. By integrating these techniques into their lives, women can navigate menopause with greater ease, confidence, and well-being. These holistic approaches provide a pathway to not only surviving but thriving during this transformative period.

Aromatherapy and Other Holistic Approaches

Aromatherapy and holistic approaches have become the chic, go-to remedies for alleviating the symptoms of menopause, offering a stylish complement to conventional medical treatments. These natural therapies focus on the exquisite interplay between mind and body, utilizing the pure essence of nature to enhance health and well-being.

Aromatherapy, the art of using essential oils derived from plants, stands out as a particularly effective way to soothe menopausal symptoms. These fragrant elixirs can be experienced through various luxurious methods such as inhalation, massage, and indulgent baths. Imagine the calming embrace of lavender oil, renowned for its tranquil properties that ease anxiety, enhance sleep, and stabilize mood swings. Clary sage, another favored essential oil, is celebrated for its ability to balance hormones and diminish hot flashes, while peppermint oil, with its invigorating coolness, offers relief from those notorious night sweats. The chicest application method might involve a sophisticated diffuser that releases a continuous stream of scent, filling the air with therapeutic goodness. Alternatively, blending essential oils with a carrier oil for a divine massage can melt away muscle tension and promote relaxation.

Beyond the allure of aromatherapy, holistic approaches to menopause include the timeless practice of acupuncture. This ancient Chinese technique, involving the delicate insertion of fine needles into strategic points on the body, is lauded for reducing the frequency and intensity of hot flashes, improving sleep quality, and alleviating menopause-related anxiety and depression. The magic of acupuncture lies in its ability to harmonize the body's energy flow, or "qi," restoring balance and tranquility. Many women find acupuncture a sophisticated addition to their wellness regime, offering relief from both physical and emotional symptoms sans the side effects of conventional medications.

Herbal medicine, another pillar of holistic wellness, provides potent remedies for menopausal discomforts. Time-honored herbs like black cohosh, red clover, and dong quai have long been used to manage symptoms such as hot flashes, night sweats, and mood swings. Black cohosh, in particular, is well-researched and shown to significantly reduce hot flash severity. Red clover, rich in phytoestrogens, mimics estrogen in the body, soothing the effects of estrogen deficiency. However, it's imperative to consult with a healthcare provider before embarking on any herbal regimen to ensure safety and avoid potential drug interactions.

Nutrition also plays a pivotal role in a holistic menopause strategy. A diet brimming with phytoestrogens—think soy products, flaxseeds, and legumes—can help counteract the decline in estrogen. Omega-3 fatty acids, found in fish oil, chia seeds, and walnuts, are lauded for their anti-inflammatory properties and support of mental health. Incorporating these nutritional powerhouses into daily meals can naturally manage symptoms and elevate overall wellness.

Mind-body practices such as yoga, tai chi, and mindfulness meditation are also essential components of holistic menopause management. These practices offer a refined blend of physical movement, breath control, and meditation, fostering relaxation, reducing stress, and uplifting mood. Regular engagement in yoga or tai chi enhances flexibility, strength, and balance, which become increasingly vital with age.

Moreover, lifestyle modifications such as maintaining a consistent exercise routine, ensuring adequate sleep, and employing stress-reduction techniques are indispensable to a holistic menopause approach. Regular physical activity harmonizes hormone levels, boosts mood, and helps maintain a healthy weight. Prioritizing restful sleep and incorporating relaxation techniques like deep breathing, progressive muscle relaxation, and guided imagery can significantly mitigate menopausal symptoms.

Aromatherapy and other holistic approaches offer an elegant toolkit for managing the myriad symptoms of menopause. By embracing these natural therapies, women can experience relief from physical and emotional discomforts, ultimately enhancing their quality of life during this transformative period. These approaches highlight the importance of balance, self-care, and the intricate mind-body connection, providing a sophisticated framework for navigating menopause with grace and resilience.

CHAPTER 4

Long-Term Health And Wellness

Bone Health and Osteoporosis Prevention

Importance of Calcium and Vitamin D

Calcium and Vitamin D are essential nutrients, especially for women navigating the transformative journey of menopause. Their significance is monumental, as these power duo nutrients are foundational in safeguarding bone health and warding off osteoporosis, a condition that becomes more prevalent due to the hormonal shifts of menopause.

Calcium, a vital mineral, is indispensable for a multitude of bodily functions, including muscle contraction, blood clotting, and nerve transmission. However, its most glamorous role is maintaining bone health. A staggering 99% of the body's calcium resides in bones and teeth, providing them with structure and strength. During menopause, the decline in estrogen levels accelerates bone loss, heightening the risk of osteoporosis—a condition characterized by brittle, fragile bones. Ensuring an ample intake of calcium is crucial to mitigate this risk by enhancing bone density and strength. Fabulous dietary sources of calcium include dairy delights like milk, cheese, and yogurt, as well as leafy green vegetables, nuts, seeds, and fortified foods. For those who find it challenging to meet their calcium needs through diet alone, supplements can be a chic alternative, but it's essential to consult a healthcare provider to determine the appropriate dosage and avoid any unwanted side effects.

Vitamin D, often hailed as the "sunshine vitamin," is equally vital for calcium absorption and bone health. Without sufficient vitamin D, the body cannot absorb calcium effectively, no matter how rich the diet is in this mineral. Vitamin D also supports immune function, reduces inflammation, and enhances muscle health. During menopause, maintaining adequate levels of vitamin D is particularly important as it helps combat the accelerated bone loss linked to declining estrogen levels. The primary source of vitamin D is sunlight exposure, but factors like geographic location, skin pigmentation, sunscreen use, and age can affect the body's ability to synthesize vitamin D from sunlight. Therefore, obtaining vitamin D from dietary sources and supplements is often necessary. Foods rich in vitamin D include fatty fish such as salmon and mackerel, fortified dairy and plant-based milks, egg yolks, and certain mushrooms.

The harmonious relationship between calcium and vitamin D is crucial for optimal bone health. Vitamin D enhances the absorption of calcium in the intestines, ensuring adequate serum calcium levels necessary for bone mineralization. Without sufficient vitamin D, the body may resort to mobilizing calcium from the bones to maintain blood calcium levels, leading to weakened bones and a higher risk of fractures. Thus, ensuring adequate intake of both nutrients is essential for minimizing bone loss and maintaining bone strength during and after menopause.

Beyond bone health, the benefits of calcium and vitamin D extend to other aspects of wellness. Adequate calcium intake has been associated with a reduced risk of hypertension and colorectal cancer. Vitamin D, meanwhile, has been linked to a lower risk of autoimmune diseases, certain cancers, and cardiovascular diseases. It also supports muscle function, which is particularly vital for maintaining mobility and preventing falls in older adults.

However, it's essential to note that excessive intake of calcium and vitamin D can have adverse effects. High calcium intake, particularly from supplements, can lead to kidney stones and impaired absorption of other essential minerals. Excessive vitamin D can result in hypercalcemia, characterized by elevated blood calcium levels, which can cause vascular and tissue calcification, kidney damage, and cardiovascular issues. Therefore, balancing adequate intake with potential risks is crucial, ideally under the guidance of a healthcare provider.

Calcium and vitamin D are indispensable for maintaining bone health and preventing osteoporosis, especially during and after menopause. Their combined roles in promoting calcium absorption and bone mineralization underscore the importance of ensuring sufficient intake through diet, sunlight exposure, and supplements if necessary. By prioritizing these nutrients, women can elegantly manage the challenges of menopause, supporting overall health and reducing the risk of long-term complications.

Exercises for Bone Strength

Exercise plays an indispensable role in maintaining bone strength, especially for women navigating the journey of menopause. As estrogen levels decline during this phase, the risk of osteoporosis and fractures increases. By engaging in targeted exercises, women can counteract these risks, promoting bone density, improving balance, and enhancing overall musculoskeletal health. Mastering the art of effective exercise for bone strength is essential for crafting a sustainable and beneficial fitness routine.

Weight-bearing exercises are the cornerstone of bone health. These activities compel the body to work against gravity, stimulating bone formation and decelerating bone loss. Think of chic activities like brisk walking, invigorating jogging, stair climbing, and even dancing. These exercises create mechanical stress on the bones, prompting the body to produce new bone tissue. Among weight-bearing exercises, those with higher impact, such as running and jumping, are particularly potent at increasing bone density. However, for those with existing joint concerns or advanced osteoporosis, low-impact weight-bearing exercises like brisk walking or using an elliptical machine provide a gentle yet effective alternative.

Resistance training, the elegant cousin of strength training, is another vital element of a bone-strengthening regimen. This exercise type involves using weights, resistance bands, or body weight to create muscle contractions that stress the bones. Picture lifting free weights, mastering weight machines, or performing bodyweight exercises like push-ups and squats. The mechanical load exerted during resistance training stimulates bone-forming cells, enhancing bone mass and strength. To achieve optimal results, it's important to target all major muscle groups and gradually increase resistance over time. Exercises focusing on the back and hips, such as deadlifts and lunges, are particularly beneficial, as these areas are most vulnerable to osteoporotic fractures.

Balance and coordination exercises are essential for preventing falls, a common cause of fractures in individuals with weakened bones. Envision the grace of tai chi, yoga, and balance drills improving stability and proprioception, reducing the risk of falls and boosting overall functional ability. Tai chi, with its slow, controlled movements, enhances balance, coordination, and flexibility, contributing to a lower fall risk. Yoga, with its emphasis on strength, flexibility, and balance, offers similar benefits while also promoting mental well-being, turning exercise into a holistic experience.

Flexibility exercises, while not directly influencing bone density, play a supportive role by improving the range of motion and preventing injuries. Regular stretching keeps muscles and ligaments flexible, reducing the risk of strains and sprains. Incorporating stretches for all major muscle groups, particularly around the hips, spine, and legs, enhances mobility and supports overall physical function.

Combining various exercises into a well-rounded fitness routine yields the best results for bone health. Imagine a weekly exercise plan featuring several days of weight-bearing aerobic activities, two to three sessions of resistance training, and regular balance and flexibility exercises. Starting slowly is key, especially for those new to exercise or who have been inactive. Gradually increasing the intensity and duration of workouts ensures sustainability. Consulting with a healthcare provider or fitness professional can tailor an exercise program to individual needs, ensuring both safety and effectiveness.

Embracing a variety of exercises is essential for maintaining bone strength and overall health, particularly during and after menopause. Weight-bearing exercises, resistance training, balance activities, and flexibility exercises each contribute uniquely to bone health and should be seamlessly woven into a comprehensive fitness routine. By committing to regular physical activity, women can significantly reduce the risk of osteoporosis, enhance their quality of life, and revel in improved overall health and well-being.

Cardiovascular Health

Understanding Heart Risks

Menopause ushers in a myriad of physiological changes, one of the most profound being an elevated risk of heart disease. This heightened risk stems primarily from the decline in estrogen levels, which significantly impacts cardiovascular health. Understanding this connection is essential for women navigating this life stage, empowering them to take proactive measures to protect their heart health.

Estrogen acts as a guardian of cardiovascular health, maintaining the flexibility of blood vessels to regulate blood flow and pressure. It also enhances cholesterol profiles by boosting high-density lipoprotein (HDL) cholesterol, the "good" kind, and reducing low-density lipoprotein (LDL) cholesterol, the "bad" kind. As estrogen levels wane during menopause, these protective benefits diminish, leading to adverse cardiovascular changes. Blood vessels may stiffen, elevating blood pressure. Additionally, cholesterol levels may shift unfavorably, increasing the risk of arterial plaque buildup, known as atherosclerosis.

However, hormonal changes are not the sole culprits in increased heart risks during menopause. Several coinciding factors exacerbate cardiovascular risks. Weight gain, particularly around the abdomen, is common during menopause and poses a significant risk for heart disease. This type of fat is metabolically active, contributing to inflammation and insulin resistance, both harmful to heart health. Lifestyle changes, such as reduced physical activity and poorer dietary habits, also frequently accompany menopause, leading to conditions like hypertension, diabetes, and high cholesterol—major heart disease risk factors.

Psychological stress during menopause further impacts heart health. The transition can be emotionally taxing, with heightened anxiety, depression, and stress. Chronic stress adversely affects heart health by elevating blood pressure, increasing heart rate, and fostering unhealthy behaviors like overeating, smoking, and inactivity. These factors create a perfect storm, significantly raising the risk of cardiovascular events like heart attacks and strokes.

Despite these risks, numerous strategies can help women protect their heart health during and after menopause. Regular physical activity is one of the most potent tools against heart risks. Engaging in aerobic exercises, strength training, and flexibility routines helps maintain a healthy weight, improve cholesterol levels, lower blood pressure, and reduce stress. A heart-healthy diet is equally crucial, emphasizing fruits, vegetables, whole grains, lean proteins, and healthy fats while minimizing processed foods, sugars, and saturated fats. Omega-3 fatty acid-rich foods, such as fish, flaxseeds, and walnuts, are particularly beneficial for heart health.

Routine medical check-ups are essential for monitoring and managing heart health. Women should collaborate with healthcare providers to regularly check blood pressure, cholesterol levels, and blood sugar levels. Sometimes, medication may be necessary to manage these risk factors effectively. Hormone replacement therapy (HRT) is another consideration for managing menopausal symptoms and potentially mitigating heart risks, though it is not suitable for everyone and requires thorough discussion with a healthcare provider.

In addition to lifestyle changes, stress management techniques like mindfulness, meditation, and yoga can be incredibly beneficial. These practices help reduce stress, lower blood pressure, and enhance overall well-being. Social support is also vital during this time. Staying connected with friends, family, and support groups can provide emotional support and mitigate feelings of isolation and stress.

While menopause increases heart risks due to hormonal changes and other factors, women can take proactive steps to safeguard their heart health. Through regular physical activity, a heart-healthy diet, routine medical check-ups, and effective stress management, women can significantly reduce their risk of heart disease and maintain a healthy, active lifestyle during and after menopause. Staying informed, proactive, and engaged in their health care allows women to navigate this transition successfully and protect their heart health.

Dietary and Lifestyle Changes for Heart Health

Dietary and lifestyle changes are paramount in preserving heart health, particularly during and after menopause, when cardiovascular risks intensify due to significant hormonal shifts, especially the decline in estrogen levels. Adopting a chic, heart-healthy regimen is not only essential but can also be effortlessly stylish, allowing you to navigate this life stage with grace and vitality.

One of the most transformative dietary adjustments is embracing a balanced, heart-healthy diet. Picture your plate brimming with vibrant fruits, lush vegetables, wholesome grains, lean proteins, and luxurious healthy fats. Fruits and vegetables are not only visually appealing but also packed with essential vitamins, minerals, and antioxidants that act as heart protectors. These nutrient powerhouses also provide dietary fiber, which helps lower cholesterol and promotes a sleek digestive system. Whole grains like oats, quinoa, and whole wheat products offer fiber that keeps blood sugar levels steady and cholesterol in check.

Lean proteins are a must for maintaining heart health. Think of succulent poultry, delectable fish, hearty beans, and versatile legumes. These sources provide necessary nutrients without the saturated fats found in red meat. Indulge in fatty fish like salmon, mackerel, and sardines, which are rich in omega-3 fatty acids—perfect for reducing inflammation and lowering heart disease risk. Don't forget plant-based proteins like tofu, tempeh, and edamame, which add a chic touch to your heart-healthy menu.

Healthy fats from avocados, nuts, seeds, and olive oil should replace unhealthy fats in your diet. These fats, particularly monounsaturated and polyunsaturated, help reduce bad cholesterol levels and offer essential fatty acids for heart health. Conversely, it's essential to limit saturated and trans fats found in processed foods, fried delights, and baked goods, which can spike cholesterol levels and contribute to heart disease.

Cutting back on sodium is another critical dietary change. High sodium levels can elevate blood pressure, posing a significant heart disease risk. Limit processed foods, scrutinize food labels for sodium content, and spice up your dishes with herbs and spices instead of salt. Staying hydrated with plenty of water throughout the day also supports overall health and helps maintain optimal blood pressure levels.

Lifestyle changes are the perfect complement to dietary adjustments in your heart-health journey. Regular physical activity is your best friend. Aim for at least 150 minutes of moderate-intensity aerobic exercise per week—think brisk walking, elegant swimming, or stylish cycling. These activities help maintain a healthy weight, lower blood pressure, and improve cholesterol levels. Add strength training exercises twice a week to build muscle mass and boost metabolism, enhancing heart health further.

Managing stress is also critical for heart health. Chronic stress can lead to unhealthy behaviors like overeating, smoking, and inactivity, all of which increase cardiovascular risks. Embrace mindfulness, meditation, yoga, and deep-breathing exercises to manage stress stylishly and effectively. Prioritize beauty sleep, as poor sleep quality or insufficient rest can contribute to high blood pressure, obesity, and other heart disease risk factors.

Avoid smoking and limit alcohol consumption for a heart-healthy lifestyle. Smoking damages blood vessels, increases blood pressure, and reduces oxygen in the blood, significantly raising heart disease risk. Quitting smoking can dramatically improve cardiovascular health and reduce the risk of heart disease and stroke. Similarly, excessive alcohol consumption can lead to high blood pressure, heart failure, and other cardiovascular problems. Moderation is key—limit alcohol intake to up to one drink per day for women to mitigate these risks.

Dietary and lifestyle changes are fundamental to maintaining heart health, especially during and after menopause. Embrace a chic, balanced diet rich in fruits, vegetables, whole grains, lean proteins, and healthy fats. Combine this with regular physical activity, stress management, adequate sleep, and avoiding harmful habits. These proactive measures empower women to take control of their heart health, navigating menopause with confidence, resilience, and a touch of elegance

Sexual Health and Intimacy

Addressing Vaginal Dryness and Discomfort

Vaginal dryness and discomfort are ubiquitous challenges faced by many women during and after menopause, significantly influencing both physical comfort and emotional well-being, as well as intimate relationships. Grasping the underlying causes, recognizing the symptoms, and exploring various treatment options is essential for managing these changes with grace and efficacy.

The primary culprit behind vaginal dryness during menopause is the decline in estrogen levels. Estrogen is indispensable in preserving the health and suppleness of vaginal tissues. As estrogen levels diminish, the vaginal walls become thinner, less elastic, and more susceptible to irritation. This reduction leads to a decrease in natural lubrication, resulting in dryness, itching, and discomfort. Additionally, lower estrogen levels disrupt the vaginal pH balance, increasing vulnerability to infections and inflammation.

The severity of vaginal dryness symptoms can vary widely. Some women may experience mild discomfort, while others endure intense itching, burning, or pain. These symptoms can make daily activities such as walking or sitting uncomfortable and cause significant distress during sexual intercourse. This discomfort often leads to decreased sexual desire and intimacy, further impacting a woman's emotional and psychological well-being.

Managing vaginal dryness and discomfort involves a combination of lifestyle adjustments, over-the-counter products, and medical treatments. One of the simplest and most effective methods is the use of vaginal moisturizers and lubricants. Vaginal moisturizers, intended for regular use, maintain moisture and enhance the health of vaginal tissues, providing long-lasting relief from dryness and discomfort. Lubricants are designed for use during sexual activity to reduce friction and increase comfort. Water-based or silicone-based lubricants are recommended, as oil-based products can cause irritation and heighten the risk of infections.

Beyond over-the-counter products, several medical treatments are available. Topical estrogen therapy is among the most common and effective treatments for vaginal dryness. This involves applying estrogen directly to the vaginal area in the form of creams, tablets, or rings, which helps restore the health and elasticity of vaginal tissues, boost natural lubrication, and reduce discomfort. Given its local application, topical estrogen has minimal systemic absorption, mitigating the risk of side effects linked with hormone replacement therapy.

For women who cannot use estrogen therapy, non-hormonal alternatives exist. These include vaginal moisturizers containing hyaluronic acid, which help maintain moisture and improve the condition of vaginal tissues. Another non-hormonal option is laser therapy, which stimulates collagen production and enhances blood flow to the vaginal area, improving elasticity and lubrication.

Lifestyle modifications also play a crucial role in managing vaginal dryness. Staying hydrated by drinking plenty of water helps maintain overall body moisture, including vaginal tissues. Avoiding irritants such as scented soaps, douches, and synthetic fabrics can prevent further irritation and discomfort. Regular sexual activity, including vaginal intercourse, can help maintain vaginal health by promoting blood flow and elasticity. For women who are not sexually active, using vaginal dilators can provide similar benefits.

Addressing the emotional and psychological impacts of vaginal dryness is equally important. Open communication with a partner about symptoms and concerns can help maintain intimacy and alleviate anxiety. Seeking support from healthcare providers, therapists, or support groups can provide additional resources and coping strategies.

Vaginal dryness and discomfort, while common, are manageable symptoms of menopause. By understanding the causes and exploring a variety of treatment options, women can find effective ways to alleviate these symptoms and enhance their quality of life. Whether through lifestyle changes, over-the-counter products, or medical treatments, addressing vaginal dryness is a vital step in navigating the complexities of menopause and maintaining overall well-being.

Maintaining a Healthy Sex Life

Maintaining a vibrant sex life during menopause can present challenges due to the myriad of physical and emotional changes. However, with the right strategies, open communication, and a willingness to explore new approaches, a fulfilling sex life is absolutely attainable. Emotional intimacy and sexual satisfaction are crucial components of overall well-being and quality of life.

Menopause induces significant hormonal shifts, notably a decline in estrogen and progesterone, which can impact sexual function. Vaginal dryness, one of the most prevalent issues, can cause discomfort and pain during intercourse, leading to a decrease in libido and avoidance of sexual activity. Fortunately, various treatments can manage these symptoms effectively. Vaginal moisturizers and lubricants can alleviate dryness and enhance comfort during sex. Regular use of these products helps maintain the health of vaginal tissues and enhances sexual pleasure.

Hormone replacement therapy (HRT) is another viable option for addressing menopausal symptoms, including those affecting sexual health. HRT can help restore hormone levels, improving vaginal lubrication and elasticity, thereby reducing discomfort during sex. It is essential to discuss the benefits and risks of HRT with a healthcare provider to determine if it is the right choice for you.

Beyond physical treatments, maintaining a healthy sex life during menopause often requires open communication with your partner. Discussing changes in sexual desire, comfort levels, and any concerns fosters mutual understanding and support. This communication enhances intimacy and can lead to discovering new ways to connect sexually. Exploring different forms of sexual expression, such as massage, oral sex, or mutual masturbation, can also help maintain a satisfying sexual relationship.

Emotional well-being plays a crucial role in sexual health during menopause. Many women experience mood swings, anxiety, and depression during this time, which can affect libido and interest in sex. Addressing these emotional challenges is vital for maintaining a healthy sex life. Seeking support from a therapist or counselor can provide coping strategies and emotional support. Engaging in stress-reducing activities, such as yoga, meditation, or regular exercise, can also improve mood and energy levels, positively impacting sexual desire.

Body image can significantly influence sexual confidence during menopause. Changes in weight, skin elasticity, and overall appearance can lead to self-consciousness. Embracing these changes and focusing on body positivity can enhance sexual confidence. Partners can play a supportive role by expressing affection and appreciation, boosting self-esteem and intimacy.

Physical health is another cornerstone of a healthy sex life. Regular exercise not only improves overall fitness but also boosts energy levels, enhances mood, and increases blood flow, which can improve sexual function. A balanced diet rich in nutrients supports hormonal balance and overall health, contributing to better sexual health.

Prioritizing sleep is also crucial. Menopause can disrupt sleep patterns, leading to fatigue and reduced libido. Establishing a regular sleep routine and addressing sleep disturbances, such as hot flashes, can help improve energy levels and sexual desire.

Incorporating novelty into the sexual relationship can reignite passion and excitement. Trying new activities, positions, or settings can bring a sense of adventure and playfulness to the relationship. This can be a fun way to reconnect and rediscover each other.

Ultimately, maintaining a healthy sex life during menopause requires a multifaceted approach that addresses physical, emotional, and relational aspects. By proactively managing symptoms, fostering open communication, and prioritizing emotional and physical well-being, women can continue to enjoy a fulfilling and satisfying sex life during this stage of life. Remember, every woman's experience of menopause is unique, and finding what works best for you and your partner is key to maintaining intimacy and connection.

Communicating with Your Partner

Effective communication with your partner during menopause is paramount, as this life stage brings a myriad of physical, emotional, and psychological changes that impact both individuals in the relationship. Open, honest dialogue is essential for preserving intimacy, understanding, and mutual support. It ensures that both partners feel heard, valued, and connected, helping them navigate the complexities of menopause together.

Menopause can introduce several challenges, such as mood swings, decreased libido, and physical discomfort. These changes can create misunderstandings or feelings of isolation if not properly addressed. Therefore, it's vital to establish a safe space for open communication where both partners can express their feelings, concerns, and needs without fear of judgment. This environment of trust and openness fosters empathy and cooperation.

Educating each other about menopause is an effective strategy for enhancing communication. Understanding the biological and emotional aspects of this transition helps partners develop empathy and patience. Well-informed partners are better equipped to provide support and compassion. This shared knowledge serves as a foundation for meaningful conversations, allowing partners to discuss symptoms, fears, and expectations more comfortably.

Regular check-ins are a useful tool for maintaining open communication. These check-ins can be formal or informal, depending on what feels most natural for the couple. Setting aside time to talk about feelings, challenges, and support needs can prevent small issues from escalating into larger conflicts. It also ensures that both partners remain aligned and connected throughout the menopausal journey.

Listening is just as important as speaking. Active listening involves giving full attention to your partner, validating their feelings, and responding thoughtfully. This kind of listening shows respect and care for their experiences and perspectives. It can also provide insights into how best to support them. Sometimes, simply being there to listen can be incredibly comforting.

Non-verbal communication should not be overlooked. Body language, eye contact, and physical touch can convey understanding and affection when words might fall short. A reassuring hug or a gentle touch can speak volumes and help reinforce the emotional bond between partners.

Addressing sexual intimacy is crucial, as menopause can significantly affect this aspect of a relationship. Changes in libido, vaginal dryness, and discomfort during intercourse can create stress and distance between partners. Discussing these issues openly can lead to finding mutually agreeable solutions, such as using lubricants, exploring different forms of intimacy, or seeking medical advice if necessary. Approaching this topic with sensitivity and a willingness to adapt can help maintain a satisfying and fulfilling sexual relationship.

Expressing gratitude and appreciation is also important. Acknowledging the efforts and support of your partner can strengthen your bond and foster a positive atmosphere. Small gestures of appreciation can go a long way in maintaining emotional closeness and mutual respect.

Finally, recognizing that professional help is available if needed is key. Couples counseling can provide a neutral space to explore and address any communication issues or emotional challenges that arise during menopause. A therapist can offer guidance and tools to improve communication and strengthen the relationship.

Effective communication with your partner during menopause involves openness, empathy, and mutual support. By educating each other, actively listening, and addressing both emotional and physical needs, couples can navigate the changes brought by menopause together. This collaborative approach helps maintain a strong, loving relationship that can withstand the challenges of this transitional period.

CHAPTER 5

Practical Advice And Lifestyle Adjustments

Diet and Nutrition

Foods to Include and Avoid

Diet plays an indispensable role in managing menopause symptoms and enhancing overall well-being during this pivotal life transition. Knowing which foods to incorporate and which to avoid can significantly ease common menopausal discomforts like hot flashes, night sweats, mood swings, and weight gain, while also lowering the risk of chronic conditions such as heart disease and osteoporosis.

One of the most crucial food groups to embrace in a menopausal diet is fruits and vegetables. These nutrient-dense foods are packed with essential vitamins, minerals, and antioxidants that support overall health and fight oxidative stress. Leafy greens like spinach, kale, and broccoli are particularly beneficial due to their high calcium and magnesium content, essential for bone health. Vibrant fruits such as berries, oranges, and apples are rich in fiber and vitamin C, boosting the immune system and promoting radiant skin.

Whole grains are another dietary cornerstone for menopausal women. Choices like oats, brown rice, quinoa, and whole wheat bread provide complex carbohydrates and fiber, helping to stabilize blood sugar levels, reduce the risk of cardiovascular disease, and support digestive health. Including a variety of whole grains in your meals can also aid in weight management by promoting a feeling of fullness and sustained energy throughout the day.

Healthy fats are integral to managing menopause symptoms. Omega-3 fatty acids, found in fatty fish like salmon, mackerel, and sardines, as well as in flaxseeds, chia seeds, and walnuts, offer anti-inflammatory benefits and support heart health. These fats can help diminish the frequency and severity of hot flashes and bolster brain function, which is especially beneficial in addressing menopause-related mood swings and cognitive changes.

Protein is a vital nutrient during menopause, essential for maintaining muscle mass and supporting metabolic health. Opt for lean protein sources such as chicken, turkey, tofu, legumes, and low-fat dairy products. Additionally, soy-based foods like tofu, tempeh, and edamame are advantageous due to their phytoestrogen content—plant compounds that mimic estrogen in the body and can help balance hormone levels, potentially alleviating hot flashes and other menopausal symptoms.

Conversely, certain foods should be limited or avoided to manage menopause symptoms effectively. Highly processed foods, often laden with added sugars, unhealthy fats, and sodium, can worsen symptoms like weight gain, bloating, and mood swings. Sugary snacks, sugary beverages, and refined carbohydrates such as white bread and pastries can cause rapid blood sugar spikes and crashes, leading to energy fluctuations and irritability.

Caffeine and alcohol should also be consumed in moderation, as they can trigger hot flashes and disturb sleep patterns. Reducing the intake of caffeinated beverages like coffee, tea, and soda, along with limiting alcohol consumption, can help mitigate these effects. Even if eliminating caffeine and alcohol entirely isn't feasible, cutting back and monitoring their impact on symptoms can still be beneficial.

It's also wise to be cautious with salty foods, as excessive sodium can lead to water retention and elevated blood pressure. Processed meats, canned soups, and salty snacks should be consumed sparingly, and flavoring food with herbs and spices instead of salt is advisable.

A balanced, nutrient-rich diet is fundamental to managing menopause symptoms and ensuring long-term health. Incorporating a variety of fruits, vegetables, whole grains, healthy fats, and lean proteins can alleviate common menopausal symptoms and support overall well-being. Conversely, avoiding highly processed foods, excessive sugar, caffeine, alcohol, and salt can prevent exacerbating symptoms and contribute to a healthier, more comfortable transition through menopause. By making mindful dietary choices, women can navigate menopause with greater ease and improved health outcomes.

Recipes and Meal Plans for Menopause

Creating exquisite and balanced recipes tailored to the needs of menopausal women can significantly alleviate common symptoms and promote overall well-being. Menopause brings about hormonal fluctuations that can lead to various physical and emotional changes, including hot flashes, mood swings, weight gain, and bone density loss. A well-structured meal plan that incorporates specific nutrients can help mitigate these symptoms and support a healthy transition through menopause.

Breakfast: Energize Your Morning

Start your day with a nutrient-rich breakfast that sets the tone for vitality and balance. Consider a chic smoothie crafted with leafy greens like spinach or kale, bursting with calcium and magnesium to fortify bone health. Add a medley of vibrant berries for a dose of antioxidants and fiber, promoting heart health and aiding digestion. To keep your blood sugar levels stable and maintain muscle mass, blend in Greek yogurt or a scoop of plant-based protein powder.

Recipe Idea: Spinach and Berry Smoothie

Handful of spinach

1/2 cup mixed berries

1/2 cup Greek yogurt

1 scoop plant-based protein powder

1 cup almond milk

Blend until smooth and enjoy!

Lunch: Chic and Nutritious

For lunch, a balanced salad can be both satisfying and beneficial. Assemble a colorful array of vegetables like bell peppers, tomatoes, cucumbers, and carrots to ensure a broad spectrum of vitamins and minerals. Top your salad with grilled chicken, tofu, or chickpeas for a protein boost, and sprinkle with flaxseeds or chia seeds, rich in omega-3 fatty acids. These seeds have anti-inflammatory properties and can help reduce the frequency and severity of hot flashes. Dress your salad with a light vinaigrette made from olive oil and lemon juice for a touch of healthy fats and a refreshing flavor.

Recipe Idea: Omega-3 Power Salad

Mixed greens

1/2 cup cherry tomatoes

1/2 cup sliced cucumbers

1/2 bell pepper, sliced

1/2 cup chickpeas

1 tbsp flaxseeds

Olive oil and lemon juice vinaigrette

Toss and savor!

Dinner: Sophisticated and Satisfying

Dinner should be a harmonious blend of lean proteins, whole grains, and vibrant vegetables. A baked salmon fillet accompanied by a quinoa and vegetable stir-fry is an elegant choice. Salmon is an excellent source of omega-3 fatty acids and vitamin D, crucial for heart health and bone strength. Quinoa offers a complete protein and is rich in fiber, aiding digestion and helping maintain a healthy weight. Including a variety of vegetables like broccoli, bell peppers, and snap peas ensures a robust intake of essential vitamins and minerals.

Recipe Idea: Baked Salmon with Quinoa Stir-Fry

1 salmon fillet

1 cup cooked quinoa

1/2 cup broccoli florets

1/2 cup bell pepper slices

1/2 cup snap peas

Season salmon with herbs and bake at 375°F for 20 mi

Stir-fry vegetables with quinoa, olive oil, and a pinch

Plate and enjoy a gourmet dinner!

Snacks: Nourishing and Delightful

Snacks between meals should be both nourishing and enjoyable. A small handful of almonds or walnuts provides a quick source of protein and healthy fats. Pairing nuts with a piece of fruit, such as an apple or banana, adds fiber and vitamins, keeping your energy levels steady throughout the day. Greek yogurt with a drizzle of honey and a sprinkle of flaxseeds combines probiotics for gut health, protein, and omega-3s.

Recipe Idea: Greek Yogurt Delight

1/2 cup Greek yogurt

Drizzle of honey

1 tbsp flaxseeds

Mix and indulge!

Embrace Phytoestrogens and Herbal Teas

Incorporating phytoestrogen-rich foods into your diet can help balance hormone levels naturally. Soy-based products like tofu, tempeh, and edamame contain isoflavones, which mimic estrogen in the body and can alleviate menopausal symptoms. Herbal teas, such as chamomile or peppermint, are soothing and can help with sleep disturbances, a common issue during menopause.

Sample Meal Plan: A Day of Elegance

Breakfast: Spinach and berry smoothie

Lunch: Mixed vegetable and chickpea salad

Snack: Handful of almonds and an apple

Dinner: Baked salmon fillet with quinoa and a variety of steamed vegetables

Evening: A soothing cup of chamomile tea to promote relaxation and restful sleep

By carefully planning meals and incorporating a variety of nutrient-dense foods, you can address the unique nutritional needs of menopausal women. This approach not only helps manage symptoms but also supports overall health and well-being, making the journey through menopause smoother and more comfortable.

The Role of Phytoestrogens and Other Nutrients

The role of phytoestrogens and other essential nutrients in managing menopause symptoms has recently garnered significant attention. Phytoestrogens, plant-derived compounds that mimic estrogen's effects, offer a natural solution for women navigating the hormonal shifts of menopause. Embracing these natural elements and integrating them into a sophisticated, balanced diet can provide relief from common symptoms and enhance overall well-being.

Phytoestrogens are abundant in foods like soy products—think tofu, tempeh, and edamame. These soy delicacies contain isoflavones, a type of phytoestrogen known for its ability to bind to estrogen receptors, effectively alleviating menopause symptoms such as hot flashes, night sweats, and mood swings. Incorporating soy into your daily diet can harmonize hormonal imbalances, leading to a smoother menopausal experience.

Beyond soy, other foods rich in phytoestrogens include flaxseeds, sesame seeds, and select legumes. Flaxseeds are particularly remarkable due to their high lignan content. These versatile seeds can effortlessly be added to smoothies, yogurt, or salads. Regular consumption of flaxseeds not only supplies phytoestrogens but also offers dietary fiber and omega-3 fatty acids, which are vital for heart health and reducing inflammation.

In addition to phytoestrogens, other nutrients play pivotal roles in managing menopause symptoms and sustaining overall health. Calcium and vitamin D are indispensable for bone health, especially as declining estrogen levels can lead to reduced bone density and heightened osteoporosis risk. Dairy products, leafy greens, and fortified foods are excellent calcium sources, while vitamin D can be sourced from sunlight, fatty fish, and fortified foods. Ensuring sufficient intake of these nutrients is crucial for mitigating bone loss and minimizing fracture risks.

Magnesium, known for its mood-regulating, sleep-enhancing, and muscle-relaxing properties, is another essential nutrient during menopause. Nuts, seeds, whole grains, and leafy greens are rich in magnesium. Adequate magnesium intake can alleviate insomnia, reduce mood swings and anxiety, fostering a more stable emotional state during menopause.

B vitamins, particularly B6 and B12, are vital for maintaining energy and cognitive function. Whole grains, lean meats, eggs, and dairy products are excellent sources. Including these foods in your diet can combat fatigue and brain fog, common menopausal complaints.

Omega-3 fatty acids, found in fatty fish like salmon, mackerel, and sardines, as well as in flaxseeds and walnuts, are celebrated for their anti-inflammatory properties and heart health benefits. These fatty acids can lower cardiovascular disease risk, which becomes more significant post-menopause as estrogen's protective effects wane. Additionally, omega-3s enhance mood and cognitive function, offering a comprehensive approach to managing menopause symptoms.

Antioxidants, found in an array of fruits and vegetables, protect the body from oxidative stress and inflammation. Vitamins C and E, beta-carotene, and selenium are potent antioxidants that bolster overall health and alleviate menopause symptoms. A diet abundant in colorful fruits and vegetables ensures a steady supply of these vital nutrients, promoting vitality and well-being.

In summary, incorporating phytoestrogens and other crucial nutrients into your diet can significantly benefit women undergoing menopause. These nutrients help balance hormones, maintain bone health, support mood and cognitive function, and reduce chronic disease risks. By focusing on a nutrient-rich diet, women can gracefully navigate menopause and enhance their quality of life during this transformative phase.

Exercise and Fitness

Designing a Fitness Routine for Menopause

Crafting an exquisite fitness routine for menopause is essential to navigating the physical and emotional changes that accompany this natural phase of life. Menopause introduces hormonal fluctuations that can lead to weight gain, muscle loss, decreased bone density, and mood swings. A meticulously balanced exercise program can mitigate these symptoms, elevate overall health, and enhance quality of life. Designing a sophisticated and effective fitness regimen involves blending various types of physical activities, acknowledging the body's evolving needs, and maintaining steadfast consistency.

Cardiovascular exercise remains the epitome of any fitness routine, especially for menopausal women. Engaging in aerobic activities like brisk walking, jogging, swimming, or cycling not only bolsters heart health but also revs up metabolism and aids in weight management. As metabolism decelerates during menopause, weight gain becomes more probable. Regular cardio sessions increase calorie expenditure and improve cardiovascular endurance. Strive for at least 150 minutes of moderate-intensity or 75 minutes of vigorous aerobic exercise weekly. This regimen helps manage weight while simultaneously diminishing the risk of heart disease, which becomes more prevalent post-menopause.

Strength training is another indispensable element of a menopausal fitness routine. With declining estrogen levels, muscle mass and bone density diminish. Incorporating resistance exercises such as weight lifting, bodyweight routines, or resistance band workouts is vital for building and preserving muscle mass, fortifying bones, and enhancing metabolic rate. Ensure your strength training targets all major muscle groups, including the legs, back, chest, arms, and core. Aim for strength training sessions two to three times per week to safeguard muscle and bone health while boosting overall strength and functionality.

Flexibility and balance exercises hold equal importance during menopause. Hormonal shifts can compromise joint health and elevate fall risks due to reduced bone density. Practices like yoga, Pilates, and tai chi enhance flexibility, bolster balance, and encourage mindfulness. These activities alleviate stiffness, improve posture, and ease joint discomfort. Furthermore, the meditative qualities of yoga and tai chi offer profound mental health benefits, reducing stress and anxiety, elevating mood, and enhancing sleep quality.

Incorporating high-intensity interval training (HIIT) can be particularly advantageous for menopausal women. HIIT consists of brief, intense exercise bursts interspersed with rest or low-intensity periods. This training method effectively boosts metabolism, improves cardiovascular health, and promotes fat loss. However, caution is imperative, especially for beginners or those with existing health conditions. Consulting a fitness professional ensures HIIT workouts are safe and tailored to individual fitness levels.

Consistency is the hallmark of any successful fitness routine, and this is particularly true for menopausal women. Establish a regular exercise schedule and adhere to it to sustain the benefits of physical activity. It is also crucial to listen to your body and adjust the routine as necessary. Some days may call for rest or lighter workouts, while others may accommodate more intense sessions. Flexibility and adaptability in your fitness routine ensure long-term adherence and success.

Beyond the physical advantages, a well-curated fitness routine offers substantial mental and emotional benefits. Exercise stimulates endorphin release, naturally lifting the mood and combating mood swings, anxiety, and depression commonly associated with menopause. Regular physical activity also promotes improved sleep, often disrupted by menopausal symptoms like night sweats.

Designing an elegant fitness routine for menopause requires a balanced blend of cardiovascular exercise, strength training, flexibility, and balance activities, and potentially HIIT. Consistency, adaptability, and a focus on holistic health are paramount for managing menopausal symptoms and enhancing overall well-being. By prioritizing fitness, menopausal women can gracefully navigate this life stage with vitality and confidence.

Benefits of Strength Training and Aerobic Exercise

Strength training and aerobic exercise each bring distinct and profound benefits, especially for women experiencing menopause. As the body undergoes substantial hormonal shifts during this time, maintaining an active lifestyle becomes paramount in managing symptoms and enhancing overall health. By seamlessly blending strength training and aerobic exercise, women can effectively address the various physical and mental challenges associated with menopause, ultimately achieving a higher quality of life.

Strength training, which includes activities like weight lifting, resistance band workouts, and bodyweight exercises, is indispensable for preserving and building muscle mass. With the decline in estrogen levels during menopause, muscle mass and bone density can decrease. Regular strength training helps counteract these effects by stimulating muscle growth and fortifying bone strength. This not only boosts physical strength and endurance but also reduces the risk of osteoporosis, a prevalent concern for post-menopausal women. Stronger muscles and bones lead to better stability and a decreased likelihood of falls and fractures, which is crucial for maintaining independence and mobility as one ages.

Moreover, strength training offers significant metabolic benefits. Muscle tissue is more metabolically active than fat tissue, so increasing muscle mass helps elevate the body's resting metabolic rate. This means that even at rest, the body burns more calories, aiding in weight management—a common challenge during menopause due to a slowing metabolism. Strength training can also improve insulin sensitivity, which helps regulate blood sugar levels and diminish the risk of type 2 diabetes.

On the other hand, aerobic exercise focuses on enhancing cardiovascular health. Activities such as walking, running, cycling, swimming, and dancing raise the heart rate and improve the cardiovascular system's efficiency. For menopausal women, regular aerobic exercise is particularly beneficial in reducing the risk of heart disease, which becomes more pronounced after menopause. By bolstering heart health, aerobic exercise helps lower blood pressure, reduce cholesterol levels, and improve overall cardiovascular function. This form of exercise also aids in weight management by burning calories and enhancing metabolic health.

Beyond its physical benefits, aerobic exercise plays a crucial role in mental well-being. Exercise-induced endorphins act as natural mood enhancers, helping to alleviate symptoms of depression and anxiety, which often intensify during menopause. Regular aerobic activity can also improve sleep quality, reduce stress, and uplift overall mood. For many women, this translates to better emotional stability and a heightened sense of well-being.

Combining strength training with aerobic exercise offers a holistic approach to fitness that maximizes benefits. While strength training builds muscle and strengthens bones, aerobic exercise boosts cardiovascular health and mental well-being. Together, they create a balanced workout regimen that addresses the multifaceted challenges of menopause.

Consistency is key to reaping the full benefits of these exercises. It is important to integrate both types of workouts into a regular fitness routine, aiming for at least two to three strength training sessions per week and 150 minutes of moderate-intensity aerobic exercise. By doing so, menopausal women can significantly enhance their physical health, manage weight, reduce the risk of chronic diseases, and boost mental and emotional well-being.

The advantages of strength training and aerobic exercise are extensive and crucial, particularly for menopausal women. Strength training aids in building muscle mass, improving bone density, and boosting metabolism, while aerobic exercise enhances cardiovascular health, aids in weight management, and promotes mental well-being. By incorporating both forms of exercise into a consistent fitness routine, women can effectively manage menopause symptoms and enjoy a healthier, more fulfilling life.

Mind-Body Exercises: Yoga and Pilates

Mind-body exercises like yoga and Pilates have become the epitome of holistic fitness, blending physical movement with mental focus and breath control. These exercises are particularly beneficial for women experiencing menopause, providing a wealth of physical, emotional, and psychological advantages that help manage the multifaceted symptoms associated with this life transition.

Yoga, an ancient practice rooted in India, merges physical postures, breathing exercises, and meditation, emphasizing the unity of mind and body to foster balance and inner peace. For menopausal women, yoga serves as a potent remedy for alleviating hot flashes, mood swings, and sleep disturbances. The physical postures, or asanas, enhance flexibility, strength, and balance—key factors as muscle mass and bone density tend to decline with age. Poses such as Warrior, Tree, and Bridge fortify the core and lower body, bolstering stability and mitigating the risk of falls.

In addition to physical benefits, yoga's emphasis on breath control, or pranayama, is remarkably effective in managing stress and anxiety. Deep, rhythmic breathing activates the parasympathetic nervous system, promoting relaxation and curbing the production of cortisol, a stress hormone. This is especially crucial during menopause when hormonal fluctuations can heighten stress and anxiety. Regular yoga practice nurtures mindfulness and present-moment awareness, encouraging a positive and accepting mindset toward bodily changes.

Pilates, conceived by Joseph Pilates in the early 20th century, prioritizes core strength, flexibility, and overall body awareness. While it shares the mind-body connection with yoga, Pilates focuses on controlled movements and precision, often utilizing specialized equipment like the Reformer or performed on a mat with body weight. For menopausal women, Pilates is particularly advantageous in fortifying pelvic floor muscles, which can weaken due to hormonal changes. Strong pelvic floor muscles help prevent urinary incontinence, a common menopausal concern.

Pilates also enhances posture and alignment, reducing the risk of back pain and other musculoskeletal issues. Controlled movements improve muscle tone and joint mobility, promoting a greater range of motion and flexibility essential for maintaining functional fitness and independence with age. Moreover, Pilates' focus on breath control and concentration aids in stress reduction and mental clarity, countering the cognitive fog often associated with menopause.

Both yoga and Pilates foster a supportive community atmosphere, providing social interaction and a sense of belonging that can be uplifting during menopause's emotional fluctuations. Participating in group classes or online communities offers a platform for sharing experiences and coping strategies, reducing feelings of isolation and promoting a positive outlook.

Incorporating yoga and Pilates into a regular fitness regimen offers a holistic approach to managing menopause symptoms. These practices not only enhance physical fitness by improving strength, flexibility, and balance but also promote mental well-being through stress reduction, mindfulness, and emotional resilience. For many women, yoga and Pilates become indispensable components of their self-care routine, empowering them to navigate menopause with greater ease and confidence.

Mind-body exercises like yoga and Pilates present a comprehensive approach to health and wellness, particularly beneficial for menopausal women. By integrating these practices into daily life, women can effectively manage physical symptoms, alleviate stress and anxiety, and elevate their overall quality of life. The holistic nature of yoga and Pilates makes them invaluable tools for fostering a balanced and harmonious approach to the challenges of menopause.

Sleep and Relaxation

Tips for Improving Sleep Quality

Enhancing sleep quality is paramount for maintaining overall health and well-being, especially during menopause, when hormonal fluctuations can significantly disrupt sleep patterns. Many women face insomnia, frequent awakenings, and restless nights, exacerbating other menopausal symptoms such as mood swings, fatigue, and cognitive difficulties. Here are some chic and effective strategies to elevate your sleep quality during this transformative phase.

Establish a Consistent Sleep Schedule: Cultivate a regular sleep routine by going to bed and waking up at the same time each day. This consistency helps regulate your body's internal clock, facilitating a natural sleep-wake cycle. Maintain this schedule even on weekends to reinforce your body's rhythm. Indulge in a pre-sleep ritual, such as reading a captivating book, luxuriating in a warm bath, or practicing relaxation techniques like deep breathing or meditation, to signal to your body that it's time to unwind.

Create a Sleep-Inducing Environment: Transform your bedroom into a serene sanctuary dedicated to rest and relaxation. Ensure the room is dark, quiet, and cool to enhance sleep quality. Utilize blackout curtains, white noise machines, or earplugs to eliminate disruptive light and sounds. Keep the bedroom temperature comfortably cool, ideally between 60-67 degrees Fahrenheit, to align with the body's natural drop in temperature during sleep.

Limit Screen Exposure: The blue light emitted by phones, tablets, computers, and televisions can hinder melatonin production, the hormone that regulates sleep. Turn off electronic devices at least an hour before bed. Opt for calming activities like reading a physical book, journaling, or listening to soothing music to create a more conducive environment for falling asleep.

Mind Your Dietary Habits: Be mindful of your evening dietary choices. Consuming heavy meals, caffeine, or alcohol close to bedtime can disrupt sleep. Caffeine, found in coffee, tea, and many sodas, can linger in your system for hours, making it challenging to fall asleep. While alcohol may initially induce drowsiness, it can interfere with deeper sleep stages, leading to fragmented rest. Opt for lighter meals in the evening and avoid caffeine and alcohol several hours before bedtime.

Incorporate Regular Physical Activity: Regular exercise is beneficial for sleep, but timing is crucial. Avoid vigorous workouts close to bedtime, as they can be stimulating. Aim to finish exercising at least a few hours before bed. Evening gentle exercises, such as yoga or stretching, can promote relaxation and improve sleep quality.

Manage Stress and Anxiety: Stress and anxiety can keep your mind active, making it difficult to relax and fall asleep. Embrace stress-reducing techniques like mindfulness meditation, progressive muscle relaxation, or guided imagery to calm your mind. Keeping a worry journal to jot down concerns before bed can help clear your mind and reduce nighttime anxiety.

Seek Professional Help if Needed: If sleep disturbances persist, consider seeking professional assistance. A healthcare provider can evaluate underlying conditions such as sleep apnea or restless legs syndrome, which may require specific treatments. Cognitive-behavioral therapy for insomnia (CBT-I) can also be highly effective for chronic sleep issues.

Elevate Your Sleep Quality: Improving sleep quality requires a holistic approach, incorporating lifestyle changes, environmental adjustments, and stress management techniques. By embracing these strategies, women navigating menopause can achieve more restful and restorative sleep, essential for overall health and well-being during this significant life transition.

By adopting these elegant and effective sleep-enhancing practices, you can navigate menopause with grace, ensuring that each night is as restful and rejuvenating as possible.

Stress Management Techniques

Stress management techniques are essential for maintaining overall well-being, especially during challenging phases like menopause. The hormonal fluctuations characteristic of menopause can amplify stress, making it crucial to adopt effective strategies to manage it. Embracing sophisticated and chic stress management techniques can lead to improved physical health, emotional stability, and a higher quality of life.

Embrace Mindfulness Meditation: Mindfulness meditation is a refined practice that encourages staying present in the moment. This elegant technique helps reduce the tendency to dwell on past events or worry about the future. Simple yet profound practices such as deep breathing exercises, progressive muscle relaxation, and guided imagery help calm the mind, lower blood pressure, and decrease cortisol levels. Regular mindfulness meditation can transform how the brain responds to stress, promoting serenity and composure.

Engage in Physical Activity: Exercise is a powerful antidote to stress. It releases endorphins, the body's natural mood elevators. Indulge in activities such as walking, jogging, swimming, or yoga to experience the holistic benefits. Yoga, in particular, combines graceful physical postures with breath control and meditation, making it a sophisticated approach to stress reduction. The fluid movements release tension, while focused breathing and meditation calm the mind. Regular exercise not only manages stress but also enhances sleep, self-esteem, and overall physical health.

Maintain Social Connections: Cultivate a vibrant social life by sharing experiences and feelings with friends, family, or support groups. Engaging in heartfelt conversations with those who understand your journey can provide emotional support and diminish feelings of isolation. Participating in social activities, whether through clubs, classes, or community groups, fosters a sense of community and belonging, vital for emotional well-being.

Master Time Management: Sophisticated time management skills are essential in reducing stress. Prioritize tasks, set realistic goals, and break tasks into manageable steps to prevent overwhelm. Learn to say no and delegate tasks when necessary. Craft a balanced schedule that includes time for work, relaxation, and joyful activities. A well-organized plan provides a sense of control, reducing the chaos that often leads to stress.

Indulge in Hobbies and Leisure Activities: Engaging in hobbies such as gardening, reading, painting, or playing a musical instrument offers a delightful escape from daily stresses. These activities promote a sense of accomplishment and relaxation, providing a much-needed break. Dedicate time to pursuits that bring joy and fulfillment, significantly reducing stress levels.

Prioritize Sleep: Elegant sleep hygiene practices are vital for stress management. Lack of sleep exacerbates stress and negatively impacts overall health. Establish a regular sleep routine, create a restful environment, and avoid stimulants like caffeine before bedtime. Ensuring the body and mind are well-rested equips you to handle stress with grace.

Nourish with Nutrition: A balanced diet is paramount in managing stress. Indulge in a diet rich in fruits, vegetables, whole grains, and lean proteins to enhance energy levels and mood. Avoid excessive sugar and caffeine to prevent mood swings and energy crashes. Staying hydrated and moderating alcohol intake are essential for maintaining a stable mood and overall health.

Seek Professional Guidance: When stress becomes overwhelming, seeking professional help is a wise decision. Consult with a mental health professional to explore therapies such as cognitive-behavioral therapy (CBT), which offers strategies to change negative thought patterns and behaviors. A therapist can help identify stress sources and develop personalized coping strategies, ensuring you navigate menopause with sophistication and resilience.

Incorporating these stress management techniques into your daily routine will lead to significant improvements in emotional and physical well-being. By actively managing stress, you can navigate the challenges of menopause with elegance and enjoy a higher quality of life.

Relaxation Exercises and Practices

In the sophisticated world of wellness, relaxation exercises are indispensable for preserving both mental and physical health, particularly during stressful periods or transitional phases like menopause. These luxurious techniques not only reduce stress but also lower blood pressure and enhance overall well-being. Incorporating these relaxation practices into your daily routine can cultivate an exquisite sense of calm and balance.

Deep Breathing: Imagine a moment of serenity, achieved through the simplicity of deep breathing. This elegant technique involves inhaling slowly and deeply, filling the lungs completely, then exhaling with grace. Deep breathing activates the parasympathetic nervous system, counteracting stress and promoting tranquility. Practiced regularly, it can reduce anxiety, enhance focus, and impart a serene sense of well-being. It's a versatile practice, perfect for any setting, from a bustling cityscape to a tranquil retreat.

Progressive Muscle Relaxation (PMR): Picture the gentle release of tension through Progressive Muscle Relaxation. This refined practice involves tensing and then gradually relaxing each muscle group, from your toes to your head. PMR is ideal for those whose stress manifests physically, causing tension headaches or back pain. By systematically relaxing each muscle, this technique enhances body awareness and delivers a tangible sense of relaxation, turning stress into a distant memory.

Meditation: Elevate your mental clarity with the art of meditation. Whether it's mindfulness meditation, guided meditation, or loving-kindness meditation, each style offers its unique path to tranquility. Mindfulness meditation encourages a present-moment focus, acknowledging thoughts and feelings without judgment, which reduces stress and enhances self-awareness. Guided meditation, often led by a serene voice, provides support and direction, making it accessible for beginners. This practice cultivates a calm and emotionally balanced state, perfect for navigating life's complexities.

Yoga: Transform your routine with the holistic practice of yoga, which seamlessly blends physical postures, breath control, and meditation. The fluid movements in yoga release tension from the body, while breath control and mindfulness calm the mind. Yoga is known for reducing stress, improving flexibility, and enhancing overall health. Its adaptability to various fitness levels makes it a luxurious practice for all, turning each session into a rejuvenating escape.

Visualization: Embark on a mental retreat with visualization, a technique that involves creating calming images in the mind. This method reduces stress by shifting focus from negative thoughts to serene, positive imagery. Picture a peaceful beach or a tranquil forest, engaging all your senses to create a vivid mental escape. Visualization is particularly effective for those who respond to visual stimuli, offering a mental oasis of calm and relaxation.

Tai Chi and Qigong: Embrace the elegance of Tai Chi and Qigong, traditional Chinese practices combining slow, deliberate movements with breath control and meditation. Often described as moving meditations, these practices promote relaxation, balance, and harmony. Suitable for all ages and fitness levels, regular practice of Tai Chi and Qigong enhances physical health, reduces stress, and cultivates overall well-being.

Incorporating these relaxation exercises into your daily life can lead to significant improvements in mental and physical health. Whether through the elegance of deep breathing, the systematic relaxation of PMR, the serene focus of meditation, the holistic approach of yoga, the mental retreat of visualization, or the graceful movements of Tai Chi and Qigong, these techniques offer valuable tools for managing stress and promoting relaxation. By dedicating time each day to these practices, you can cultivate a greater sense of calm, resilience, and overall well-being, navigating life's challenges with unparalleled ease and balance.

CHAPTER 6

Emotional And Social Well - Being Mental Health and Cognitive Function

Strategies for Maintaining Cognitive Health

In the sophisticated realm of wellness, maintaining cognitive health is paramount, especially as we navigate the life transitions such as menopause. Cognitive health, the ability to think clearly, learn, and remember, can be preserved and even enhanced through a holistic approach encompassing lifestyle changes, mental exercises, and social engagement.

Exquisite Nutrition: A balanced diet is the foundation of cognitive health. Embrace a variety of nutrient-rich foods that nourish brain function and overall well-being. Diets high in antioxidants, omega-3 fatty acids, vitamins, and minerals are particularly beneficial. Indulge in leafy greens, succulent berries, nuts, seeds, and luscious fatty fish to provide essential nutrients that protect brain cells and promote neural health. Steering clear of processed foods, sugars, and saturated fats is crucial, as they can accelerate cognitive decline.

Elegant Movement: Physical activity is another cornerstone of cognitive vitality. Regular exercise enhances blood flow to the brain, nourishing cells and fostering the growth of new neural connections. Activities such as walking, swimming, cycling, and strength training have been shown to improve memory, executive function, and processing speed. Moreover, exercise reduces the risk of chronic conditions like diabetes and hypertension, which are closely linked to cognitive decline.

Intellectual Engagement: Keep your brain sharp with stimulating mental exercises. Engage in puzzles, immerse yourself in reading, master new skills, and play challenging games to stimulate the brain and maintain cognitive abilities. Activities requiring problem-solving, critical thinking, and memory retention are particularly effective. Lifelong learning, whether through courses or hobbies, keeps the brain engaged and resilient.

Social Sophistication: Social interaction is key to cognitive health. Staying socially active wards off feelings of loneliness and depression, which can negatively impact cognitive function. Regularly engaging with friends, family, and community groups provides mental stimulation and emotional support. Participating in group activities, volunteering, or joining exclusive clubs fosters social connections and keeps the brain active.

Serene Slumber: Adequate sleep is essential for cognitive health. During sleep, the brain consolidates memories and clears out toxins accumulated during the day. Poor sleep can lead to cognitive impairments such as memory loss, difficulty concentrating, and slower processing speeds. Establishing a regular sleep schedule, creating a restful environment, and practicing impeccable sleep hygiene can improve sleep quality and, in turn, cognitive function.

Zen Living: Stress management is crucial for maintaining cognitive health. Chronic stress can damage brain cells and affect areas involved in memory and learning. Techniques such as mindfulness, meditation, yoga, and deep breathing reduce stress and promote a sense of well-being. Prioritizing relaxation and self-care help maintain a balanced mental state, essential for cognitive health.

Refined Choices: Limiting alcohol consumption and avoiding smoking are also imperative for preserving cognitive function. Both alcohol and tobacco have been linked to an increased risk of cognitive decline and neurodegenerative diseases. Reducing or eliminating these substances can protect brain health and enhance overall well-being.

Vigilant Monitoring: Regular health check-ups are essential for maintaining cognitive health. Monitoring blood pressure, cholesterol levels, and blood sugar helps manage conditions that affect cognitive function. Early detection and management of health issues prevent complications that may impair cognitive abilities.

Maintaining cognitive health requires a multifaceted approach that includes a balanced diet, regular physical activity, mental stimulation, social engagement, adequate sleep, stress management, and avoiding harmful substances. By embracing these sophisticated strategies, individuals can support their cognitive function, elevate their quality of life, and reduce the risk of cognitive decline. Proactive measures taken today ensure a healthier, more vibrant brain in the future.

Dealing with Mood Swings and Anxiety

Navigating the emotional turbulence of menopause can be a daunting experience. The fluctuating levels of estrogen and progesterone contribute significantly to emotional instability. Understanding these changes and embracing effective coping strategies is essential for maintaining emotional well-being during this transformative period.

The first step in managing mood swings and anxiety is to acknowledge that these feelings are a natural part of the menopausal journey. Many women experience heightened emotions, including irritability, sadness, and anxiety, as their bodies adapt to changing hormone levels. Embracing these changes without self-judgment can alleviate the additional stress of feeling out of control or abnormal.

Elevate with Exercise: One of the most effective ways to manage mood swings is through regular physical activity. Exercise boosts endorphin levels, the body's natural mood lifters. Engaging in activities like walking, jogging, swimming, or yoga can help alleviate anxiety and depression by reducing stress hormones such as cortisol. Moreover, regular physical activity promotes better sleep, which is crucial for emotional regulation.

Nourish with Nutrition: Diet also plays a pivotal role in managing mood swings and anxiety. A balanced diet rich in whole foods, including fruits, vegetables, lean proteins, and healthy fats, stabilizes blood sugar levels and supports overall brain health. Avoiding excessive caffeine, alcohol, and sugar is key, as these can exacerbate mood swings and anxiety. Nutrients like omega-3 fatty acids, found in fish and flaxseeds, and magnesium, found in leafy greens and nuts, are known to support brain function and emotional stability.

Mindfulness and Relaxation: Practicing mindfulness and relaxation techniques can be highly beneficial. Mindfulness involves staying present and observing thoughts and feelings without judgment. Techniques such as deep breathing, progressive muscle relaxation, and guided imagery can reduce anxiety and promote calmness. Regular mindfulness meditation has been shown to decrease anxiety symptoms and improve emotional resilience.

Social Sophistication: Social support is another critical component. Connecting with friends, family, or support groups provides a sense of belonging and validation. Sharing experiences with others facing similar challenges can reduce isolation and offer practical advice and encouragement. Professional counseling or therapy can also be invaluable, providing a safe space to explore emotions and develop coping strategies.

Hormone Replacement Therapy (HRT): For some women, HRT can help manage severe mood swings and anxiety. HRT supplements the body with estrogen and progesterone to stabilize hormone levels. It's essential to discuss the potential risks and benefits with a healthcare provider to determine if it's the right choice.

Cognitive-Behavioral Therapy (CBT): CBT is another effective treatment for managing anxiety and mood swings. It focuses on identifying and changing negative thought patterns and behaviors that contribute to emotional distress. Working with a trained therapist, women can develop healthier ways of thinking and coping with stressors.

Indulge in Self-Care: Finally, self-care is paramount. Engaging in activities that bring joy and relaxation can counterbalance the stress of menopause. Whether it's reading, gardening, listening to music, or pursuing a hobby, pleasurable activities can boost mood and provide a much-needed escape from daily stressors.

Managing mood swings and anxiety during menopause requires a multifaceted approach. Embracing regular physical activity, a balanced diet, mindfulness practices, social support, and professional help can all contribute to emotional stability. By adopting these strategies, women can navigate the emotional challenges of menopause more effectively and maintain a sense of well-being during this significant life transition.

Seeking Professional Help

Seeking professional help during menopause is an essential step for women navigating the significant physical, emotional, and psychological changes that accompany this life stage. The transition into menopause, marked by a decline in reproductive hormones such as estrogen and progesterone, can lead to various symptoms, including hot flashes, mood swings, anxiety, depression, and cognitive changes. Understanding when and how to seek professional assistance can make this transition smoother and more manageable.

Your First Line of Defense: Healthcare Providers

Your primary care physician or gynecologist should be your initial point of contact when experiencing menopausal symptoms. These professionals can offer valuable insights about the menopausal transition, conduct necessary tests, and provide treatments to alleviate symptoms.

Hormone Replacement Therapy (HRT) is often discussed as a treatment option, effectively managing symptoms like hot flashes, night sweats, and vaginal dryness by supplementing the body with estrogen and progesterone. A thorough discussion about the benefits and risks associated with HRT with your healthcare provider is crucial to making an informed decision.

Mental Health Support: Psychologists and Psychiatrists

For those experiencing significant emotional or psychological distress, consulting a mental health professional is advisable. Psychologists, psychiatrists, and counselors can offer support and treatment for mood swings, anxiety, and depression associated with menopause. Cognitive-behavioral therapy (CBT) is an effective approach that helps develop coping strategies and alter negative thought patterns contributing to emotional distress. In some cases, antidepressants may be prescribed to manage severe symptoms. Mental health professionals provide a safe space to discuss fears and concerns, helping women navigate the emotional complexities of menopause.

Nutritional Guidance: Dietitians and Nutritionists

Nutritionists and dietitians play a vital role in managing menopausal symptoms through dietary interventions. These experts can design personalized nutrition plans addressing weight gain, bone health, and overall well-being. A diet rich in calcium and vitamin D is essential for maintaining bone density, while balanced nutrition can help manage weight and reduce cardiovascular risks. Nutritionists can also provide guidance on supplements and natural remedies that may alleviate menopausal symptoms.

Fitness and Physical Health: Exercise Physiologists and Trainers

Regular exercise is known to improve mood, reduce stress, and maintain a healthy weight, making exercise physiologists and fitness trainers invaluable resources. Strength training and aerobic exercises are particularly beneficial for maintaining muscle mass and cardiovascular health. These professionals can design tailored fitness programs that cater to individual needs and limitations, ensuring that women stay active and healthy during menopause.

Community and Support: Groups and Organizations

Support groups and community organizations offer an additional layer of support. Joining a support group can provide a sense of community and belonging as women share their experiences and challenges with others going through similar transitions. These groups offer emotional support, practical advice, and encouragement, making the journey through menopause less isolating.

Exploring Alternative Therapies: Acupuncture, Herbal Medicine, and More

For those seeking alternative and complementary therapies, consulting practitioners in fields such as acupuncture, herbal medicine, and naturopathy can be beneficial. These professionals offer treatments that may alleviate symptoms without the use of conventional medications. Ensuring any alternative therapies are evidence-based and discussed with your primary healthcare provider is essential to avoid potential interactions with other treatments.

Navigating menopause involves a multidisciplinary approach, addressing physical, emotional, and psychological needs. Engaging with primary care physicians, mental health professionals, nutritionists, exercise physiologists, support groups, and alternative therapy practitioners can provide comprehensive support. By leveraging the expertise of these professionals, women can navigate menopause with greater ease, ensuring a healthier and more fulfilling experience.

Building Support Networks

Importance of Family and Friends

The importance of family and friends during menopause cannot be overstated. Menopause is a transformative period in a woman's life, marked by a myriad of physical, emotional, and psychological changes. Having a strong support system comprising family and friends can make a profound difference in how a woman navigates this challenging phase. The presence of loved ones provides emotional stability, practical assistance, and a sense of belonging, all of which are crucial for overall well-being.

Emotional Anchors

Emotionally, menopause can be tumultuous. Hormonal fluctuations often lead to mood swings, irritability, and feelings of sadness or anxiety. In such moments, the empathy and understanding of family and friends become invaluable. A supportive partner who listens without judgment, children who show patience, and friends who offer a shoulder to lean on can alleviate the emotional burden. Knowing that one is not alone and that there are people who care deeply provides immense comfort.

Practical Support

Family and friends also play a critical role in providing practical support. The physical symptoms of menopause, such as hot flashes, night sweats, fatigue, and joint pain, can make daily tasks more challenging. Loved ones can step in to help with household chores, childcare, or accompany women to medical appointments. This practical assistance significantly reduces stress, allowing women to focus on self-care and managing their symptoms more effectively.

Social Connections

Social connections are vital for mental health, particularly during menopause. Engaging in social activities with friends and family offers a welcome distraction from menopausal symptoms. Whether it's a casual chat over coffee, a walk, or participating in group activities, these interactions lift spirits and promote a sense of normalcy. Social engagement helps combat feelings of isolation and loneliness, which can be exacerbated during menopause.

Shared Wisdom

Family and friends can offer valuable perspectives and advice. Sharing experiences with others who have gone through or are going through menopause can be incredibly reassuring. It's helpful to know that the challenges faced are not unique and that others have successfully navigated similar experiences. This exchange of information and tips can be empowering, leading to better coping strategies.

Partner Support

Family members, particularly partners, have a unique role in supporting a woman during menopause. Open communication is key. Understanding the physical and emotional changes that come with menopause fosters empathy and patience. Partners who educate themselves about menopause are better equipped to provide necessary support and reassurance. This understanding can strengthen relationships as both partners navigate this phase together with mutual respect and care.

Community and Support Groups

Extended social networks and community groups also offer support. Menopause support groups, whether in-person or online, provide a platform for women to connect with others facing similar challenges. These groups are a source of shared knowledge, encouragement, and solidarity. Being part of a community that understands the nuances of menopause can be immensely validating and comforting.

The importance of family and friends during menopause is multifaceted. They provide emotional support, practical help, social engagement, and valuable insights. This network of support is essential for navigating the complex landscape of menopause. The presence of caring and understanding loved ones can transform a potentially isolating and challenging period into one of growth, resilience, and strengthened relationships. Embracing the support of family and friends can make the journey through menopause a more positive and empowering experience.

Joining Support Groups and Communities

Joining support groups and communities during menopause offers a chic and essential lifeline of understanding, empathy, and practical advice. As menopause ushers in a myriad of physical, emotional, and psychological changes, the solidarity found in these groups can be profoundly comforting. Whether in-person or online, support groups provide a safe space for women to share their experiences, challenges, and coping strategies, fostering a sense of community and belonging that is both stylish and supportive.

Menopause can bring debilitating physical symptoms such as hot flashes, night sweats, fatigue, and joint pain. In these support groups, women find a platform to discuss these issues openly, free from judgment. Hearing others describe similar experiences can be reassuring, validating one's struggles and reducing feelings of isolation. Members often exchange practical tips and home remedies that have worked for them, creating a collective wisdom that benefits all.

Emotionally, menopause can feel like a rollercoaster. Mood swings, irritability, and anxiety are common due to hormonal fluctuations. Support groups provide an outlet for expressing these feelings in a non-judgmental environment. This emotional release is therapeutic, helping to alleviate the stress and anxiety associated with menopause. The empathy and understanding from others who are navigating the same phase can foster emotional resilience and a sense of calm.

Psychologically, menopause can impact self-esteem and body image. Support groups counteract negative self-perceptions by offering positive reinforcement and encouraging self-acceptance. Women share stories of how they have maintained a positive outlook and found new ways to feel confident and empowered during this transition. These narratives inspire others to see menopause not as an end, but as a glamorous new chapter filled with possibilities.

In addition to emotional support, these groups provide valuable educational resources. Discussions often include expert talks or materials on various aspects of menopause, from understanding hormonal changes to exploring treatment options. This information empowers women to make informed decisions about their health, demystifying menopause and reducing fear and uncertainty. Knowledge is power, and support groups are a stylish source of this empowerment.

Moreover, support groups foster a sense of camaraderie and friendship. The bonds formed in these groups can extend beyond meetings, creating lasting relationships built on mutual understanding and shared experiences. Social activities organized by the groups further enhance this sense of community, providing opportunities for chic socialization and fun.

Online support communities offer additional benefits, providing access to support around the clock. These platforms allow women from different geographical locations to connect, broadening the diversity of experiences and advice shared. The anonymity of online groups can also make it easier for some women to open up about their struggles, fostering honest and candid discussions.

In-person support groups offer the advantage of face-to-face interaction, which can be more personal and impactful. The physical presence of others, the ability to give and receive hugs, and the shared laughter and tears create a powerful sense of solidarity and support.

Ultimately, joining support groups and communities during menopause can significantly enhance one's quality of life. They offer emotional solace, practical advice, and a wealth of information, all within a framework of mutual support and understanding. These groups transform the menopause journey from a solitary struggle into a shared experience where women uplift and empower each other. Embracing the support of such communities can turn the challenges of menopause into opportunities for growth, resilience, and connection.

Empowerment and Self-Care

Embracing the Menopausal Transition

Embracing the menopausal transition is an invitation to reframe your perspective, deeply understand your body's changes, and commit to unparalleled self-care and acceptance. For many, menopause evokes trepidation, marked by physical discomfort, emotional fluctuations, and a sense of loss. Yet, it also holds the potential for profound personal growth, a renewed focus on well-being, and the opportunity to step into this new phase of life with grace and confidence.

The menopausal journey, or perimenopause, begins several years before menstruation ceases, lasting anywhere from a few months to over a decade. During this time, the ovaries gradually produce less estrogen, leading to symptoms such as irregular periods, hot flashes, night sweats, mood swings, and changes in sexual health. Understanding the biological underpinnings of these symptoms can help women navigate them with greater ease and acceptance.

Education is the cornerstone of embracing menopause. By demystifying the hormonal shifts driving this transition, women can transform anxiety into empowerment. Consulting healthcare professionals, reading reputable resources, and participating in educational seminars can provide valuable insights and symptom management strategies. Recognizing menopause as a natural part of aging, rather than a medical condition, shifts the focus from fear to understanding.

Self-care is paramount during this transition. It's the perfect time to prioritize physical, emotional, and mental health. Regular exercise, a balanced diet, and adequate sleep are fundamental. Physical activity, in particular, can alleviate many menopausal symptoms, helping to regulate weight, improve mood, boost energy, and reduce the risk of osteoporosis and cardiovascular disease. Incorporating relaxation techniques such as yoga, meditation, and deep-breathing exercises can manage stress and promote emotional balance.

Emotional well-being is equally crucial. Mood swings and anxiety are common due to hormonal fluctuations, and women can benefit from practices that promote emotional resilience and mental clarity. Journaling, mindfulness, and engaging in hobbies can provide fulfillment and reduce stress. Maintaining social connections is also essential; sharing experiences with friends, family, or support groups can provide solidarity and understanding. Knowing that others are navigating similar experiences can be incredibly comforting and validating.

Embracing menopause involves redefining personal identity and goals. This phase can liberate from the responsibilities and pressures of earlier life stages. With children grown and careers established, many find menopause to be a period of renewed self-discovery and freedom. It's a time to explore new interests, set new goals, and prioritize personal desires and aspirations, leading to a richer, more fulfilling life.

Moreover, menopause enhances self-awareness and self-compassion. The physical and emotional changes prompt a deeper understanding of one's body and needs. It's a time to listen to oneself, honor limits, and practice self-kindness. Accepting the necessity of seeking help—whether through medical treatments, counseling, or alternative therapies—is part of this compassionate approach.

Reframing menopause as a positive transition rather than a decline can transform the experience. Celebrating milestones, acknowledging achievements, and focusing on the strengths and wisdom gained over the years fosters pride and accomplishment. Viewing menopause as a natural progression in the journey of womanhood, filled with potential for growth and transformation, leads to a more enriching experience.

Embracing the menopausal transition requires a holistic approach that includes education, self-care, emotional well-being, and a shift in perspective. By understanding the changes occurring, prioritizing health, seeking support, and embracing new opportunities, women can navigate this phase with confidence and grace. Menopause is not just an end but a beginning—a chance to redefine oneself and embrace life with renewed vigor and wisdom.

Developing a Positive Outlook

Cultivating a positive outlook during menopause is vital for navigating this transformative life phase with elegance and resilience. While menopause can bring a variety of physical and emotional challenges, it also offers a unique opportunity for personal growth, self-discovery, and renewed focus on well-being. Embracing this change, finding meaning in the transition, and adopting strategies that foster optimism and empowerment are key to thriving during this time.

One of the initial steps in fostering a positive mindset is to shift the narrative surrounding menopause. Rather than viewing it as a decline, see it as a natural, inevitable part of aging that marks the beginning of a new chapter. Menopause signals the end of reproductive years, but it also signifies a time of transformation and reinvention. By reframing menopause as an opportunity for growth, it becomes easier to approach this phase with curiosity and acceptance.

Education plays a pivotal role in developing a positive outlook. Understanding the biological and hormonal changes that occur during menopause can demystify symptoms and alleviate anxiety. Knowledge empowers women to make informed decisions about their health and well-being. Learning about coping strategies, treatments, and lifestyle adjustments can provide a sense of control and preparedness, making the unknown less daunting and shifting the focus to proactive management and self-care.

Self-compassion is essential in cultivating a positive outlook. Menopause can evoke feelings of frustration, sadness, or grief as women adjust to changes in their bodies and lives. It's crucial to acknowledge these emotions without judgment and practice kindness towards oneself. Self-compassion means recognizing that menopause is a universal experience and seeking help and support when needed. Being gentle with oneself and allowing time to adapt can alleviate pressure and promote emotional well-being.

Connecting with others undergoing similar experiences can also enhance positivity. Sharing stories, challenges, and successes with friends, family, or support groups provides a sense of community and solidarity. Knowing that one is not alone in this journey is comforting and uplifting. Support networks offer valuable perspectives, practical advice, and emotional encouragement, making the transition feel less isolating.

Focusing on overall well-being is crucial for maintaining a positive outlook. Regular physical activity, a balanced diet, and adequate rest are foundational to feeling good physically and mentally. Exercise, in particular, improves mood, reduces stress, and boosts energy levels. Incorporating mindfulness practices such as yoga, meditation, or deep-breathing exercises can further enhance emotional resilience and promote a sense of calm and balance.

Finding joy and meaning in daily life can significantly impact one's outlook. Engaging in hobbies, pursuing new interests, and setting personal goals provides a sense of purpose and fulfillment. This phase is an excellent time to explore passions that may have been set aside due to earlier life demands. Whether it's taking up a new sport, learning a musical instrument, or traveling, these activities bring joy and enrich life.

A positive outlook also involves celebrating achievements and milestones, no matter how small. Acknowledging progress and successes, whether it's managing a symptom better or completing a personal project, reinforces a sense of capability and accomplishment. Celebrating oneself and one's journey fosters self-esteem and optimism.

Developing a positive outlook during menopause involves embracing the transition with an open heart and mind. It means reframing menopause as a time of growth, educating oneself, practicing self-compassion, connecting with others, and focusing on well-being. By finding joy, meaning, and purpose in this phase of life, women can navigate menopause with resilience, confidence, and a sense of empowerment. Menopause is not just an end but a beginning—a time to embrace new possibilities and live life to the fullest.

Self-Care Practices and Tips

Embracing self-care during the menopausal transition is essential for navigating this significant life stage with grace and resilience. Menopause brings a spectrum of physical, emotional, and psychological changes that can be challenging. By implementing effective self-care routines, women can alleviate symptoms, enhance overall well-being, and foster a sense of empowerment and control during this transformative period.

Prioritizing Physical Health

One of the most fundamental aspects of self-care during menopause is prioritizing physical health. Regular exercise is crucial as it helps manage weight, reduces stress, and boosts mood through the release of endorphins. Activities such as walking, swimming, yoga, and strength training are highly beneficial. Yoga, in particular, not only improves flexibility and strength but also promotes relaxation and reduces anxiety. Finding an enjoyable form of exercise that fits seamlessly into one's lifestyle ensures consistency and long-term commitment.

Nutritional Excellence

Nutrition plays a significant role in managing menopausal symptoms. A balanced diet rich in fruits, vegetables, whole grains, and lean proteins supports overall health and helps regulate weight. Incorporating foods high in calcium and vitamin D is essential for bone health, which can be compromised during menopause. Leafy greens, dairy products, and fortified plant-based milks are excellent sources. Additionally, phytoestrogens, found in soy, flaxseeds, and legumes, may help alleviate hormonal symptoms. Staying hydrated and limiting caffeine and alcohol can also reduce hot flashes and night sweats.

Enhancing Sleep Quality

Sleep is a critical component of self-care. Menopause often disrupts sleep patterns, leading to fatigue and irritability. Establishing a regular sleep routine can improve sleep quality. Going to bed and waking up at the same time daily, creating a restful sleep environment, and avoiding screens before bedtime are effective strategies. Practices such as deep breathing, meditation, or listening to calming music before bed can relax the mind and prepare the body for sleep.

Nurturing Emotional Well-Being

Emotional well-being is equally important during menopause. This period can bring about feelings of anxiety, sadness, or even depression. Engaging in activities that bring joy and fulfillment can counterbalance these emotions. Hobbies, creative pursuits, and spending time with loved ones provide a much-needed emotional lift. Practicing mindfulness and meditation can manage stress and promote a sense of calm. Mindfulness involves focusing on the present moment without judgment, which is particularly helpful in dealing with the emotional fluctuations of menopause.

Fostering Social Connections

Social connections are vital for emotional support and well-being. Sharing experiences and feelings with friends, family, or support groups can reduce feelings of isolation and provide a sense of community. Support groups, whether in-person or online, offer a space to connect with others who are experiencing similar challenges. This sense of solidarity is incredibly comforting and empowering.

Indulging in Personal Time

Taking time for oneself is an essential aspect of self-care. This could mean setting aside time each day for relaxation, whether it's taking a bath, reading a book, or simply enjoying a quiet moment. Self-care is about listening to one's body and mind and responding to their needs. It's about recognizing when to slow down and take a break, and not feeling guilty for prioritizing personal well-being.

Stimulating the Mind

Mental stimulation is also an important part of self-care. Engaging in activities that challenge the mind, such as puzzles, learning a new skill, or reading, keeps the brain active and healthy. This supports cognitive function and provides a sense of accomplishment and purpose.

Incorporating these self-care practices into daily life can significantly impact how one experiences menopause. By focusing on physical health, emotional well-being, and social connections, women can navigate this transition with greater ease and confidence. Self-care is not a luxury but a necessity, and taking the time to care for oneself leads to a healthier, happier, and more fulfilling life during menopause and beyond.

CHAPTER 7

Resources And Further Reading

Expert Interviews and Case Studies

Insights from Medical Professionals

Insights from medical professionals offer a critical perspective on navigating menopause with sophistication and grace. These expert insights provide evidence-based guidance and personalized care strategies, essential for understanding the intricate hormonal changes during menopause and mitigating their impact on health and well-being. Consulting with healthcare providers, such as gynecologists, endocrinologists, and primary care physicians, is key to managing this transition with poise.

Early Recognition and Symptom Management

Medical professionals emphasize the importance of recognizing menopause symptoms early. Common indicators include hot flashes, night sweats, mood swings, vaginal dryness, and irregular periods. Early identification allows for timely interventions, significantly alleviating discomfort and preventing long-term health issues. Physicians often recommend keeping a symptom diary to track changes and patterns, making medical consultations more effective.

Understanding Hormonal Changes

A primary concern during menopause is the decline in estrogen levels, affecting various bodily functions. Medical experts stress the importance of understanding these hormonal changes and their implications. Reduced estrogen can lead to decreased bone density, increasing the risk of osteoporosis. Regular bone density screenings and preventive measures, such as calcium and vitamin D supplementation, are commonly advised to maintain bone health.

Hormone Replacement Therapy (HRT)

HRT is frequently discussed among medical professionals. It involves administering estrogen or a combination of estrogen and progesterone to relieve menopausal symptoms. While HRT can be highly effective, it is not suitable for everyone. Doctors carefully evaluate the benefits and risks, considering factors such as a woman's age, health history, and risk factors for cardiovascular disease and cancer. For some, non-hormonal treatments, including lifestyle modifications and alternative therapies, may be recommended.

Lifestyle Modifications

Lifestyle changes are another focal point in professional advice for managing menopause. Physicians advocate for regular physical activity to maintain a healthy weight, improve mood, and enhance overall well-being. Exercise also supports cardiovascular health and bone density, which are critical during menopause. Additionally, dietary recommendations from medical professionals typically include a balanced diet rich in fruits, vegetables, whole grains, and lean proteins. Foods high in phytoestrogens, such as soy products, may offer some relief from hormonal symptoms.

Mental Health and Emotional Support

Mental health is crucial during menopause. Hormonal fluctuations can lead to mood swings, anxiety, and depression. Medical professionals often suggest psychological support, including counseling or therapy, to help women cope with these emotional changes. Cognitive Behavioral Therapy (CBT) is particularly effective in managing menopausal symptoms, providing strategies to address negative thoughts and behaviors.

Improving Sleep Quality

Sleep disturbances are common during menopause, and healthcare providers offer various strategies to improve sleep quality. Recommendations may include establishing a regular sleep routine, creating a comfortable sleep environment, and practicing relaxation techniques such as deep breathing or meditation before bedtime. In some cases, medical professionals may prescribe medications to address severe sleep problems.

Vaginal Health

Vaginal health is a significant concern during menopause due to decreased estrogen levels leading to dryness and discomfort. Medical professionals often recommend vaginal moisturizers or lubricants to alleviate these symptoms. In some cases, low-dose vaginal estrogen therapy may be prescribed to improve vaginal health and function.

Regular Medical Check-Ups

Regular medical check-ups are essential during menopause. These visits allow healthcare providers to monitor health changes, manage symptoms, and screen for conditions that may arise due to hormonal changes, such as cardiovascular disease or diabetes. Preventive care, including mammograms, pelvic exams, and blood pressure monitoring, is crucial for maintaining health during and after menopause.

Comprehensive, Individualized Care

The insights from medical professionals underscore the importance of a comprehensive, individualized approach to managing menopause. By combining medical advice, lifestyle modifications, and emotional support, women can navigate this transition smoothly and maintain a high quality of life. The guidance of healthcare providers ensures that women receive the care and support they need to manage the physical and emotional challenges of menopause effectively. Embracing these expert insights allows women to approach menopause with confidence, resilience, and a renewed focus on well-being.

Personal Stories from Women Who Have Thrived Through Menopause

Navigating menopause can be a daunting experience, but personal stories from women who have thrived through this transition provide inspiration and hope. These narratives illuminate the resilience, adaptability, and empowerment that can arise during this significant phase of life.

One such story is that of Maria, a 52-year-old teacher from New York. When Maria first began experiencing menopausal symptoms, she felt overwhelmed and isolated. Hot flashes disrupted her classes, and mood swings strained her relationships with colleagues and family. Determined to regain control, Maria sought advice from a gynecologist who specialized in menopause. Through hormone replacement therapy and lifestyle changes, she managed her symptoms effectively. Beyond medical intervention, Maria discovered the transformative power of yoga and mindfulness meditation. These practices not only alleviated her physical discomfort but also provided mental clarity and emotional balance. Today, Maria describes menopause as a period of personal growth, where she learned to prioritize self-care and embrace her evolving identity.

Another inspiring journey belongs to Linda, a 56-year-old business executive from California. Linda approached menopause with a proactive mindset, armed with information and a supportive network. She joined a local menopause support group where she met women experiencing similar challenges. These meetings became a lifeline, offering practical tips and emotional support. Linda also worked closely with a nutritionist to develop a diet rich in phytoestrogens, which helped mitigate her symptoms. Regular exercise, particularly strength training, became a cornerstone of her routine, boosting her energy levels and improving her mood. Linda's professional life flourished as she learned to balance her responsibilities while managing menopause, turning what could have been a tumultuous time into a testament to her resilience and determination.

Sofia, a 49-year-old artist from Texas, shares a different yet equally empowering story. Sofia struggled with severe anxiety and depression as she transitioned into menopause. These challenges threatened her creativity and zest for life. However, Sofia found solace and strength in creative expression. Painting became her therapeutic outlet, allowing her to process her emotions and channel her energy into her art. She also sought therapy and explored natural remedies like acupuncture and herbal medicine. Through this holistic approach, Sofia navigated her emotional turmoil and emerged with a renewed sense of purpose. Her artwork, deeply influenced by her menopause journey, gained recognition and connected with others experiencing similar transitions. Sofia's story highlights the power of creativity and holistic healing in transforming adversity into artistic and personal triumph.

Then there is Ellen, a 60-year-old grandmother from Florida, whose menopause journey brought her closer to her family. Ellen faced the typical symptoms of menopause but found unexpected joy in her role as a grandmother. Spending time with her grandchildren provided a sense of fulfillment and distraction from her discomfort. Ellen also became an advocate for menopause awareness, sharing her experiences with younger women in her community. She organized workshops and talks, creating a supportive space for open discussions about menopause. Ellen's journey underscores the importance of community and intergenerational support in navigating life transitions.

These personal stories demonstrate that thriving through menopause is not only possible but can lead to profound personal growth and transformation. Each woman's journey is unique, shaped by her circumstances, choices, and support systems. By sharing these narratives, we can foster a sense of solidarity and encouragement, reminding women that they are not alone. Menopause, often seen as a period of decline, can instead be a time of empowerment, resilience, and renewed purpose. These stories inspire us to embrace this transition with courage and optimism, knowing that it can lead to new beginnings and opportunities for self-discovery.

Useful Tools and Resources

Recommended Apps and Websites

In today's digital age, navigating menopause is no longer a solitary journey. There is a wealth of apps and websites designed specifically to support women through this significant life stage, offering information, community, and tools for managing symptoms. These resources are invaluable for those seeking to understand their experiences, connect with others, and find practical solutions to the challenges of menopause.

One of the most popular apps for menopause is "Caria." Formerly known as "Clio," Caria provides personalized insights into menopausal symptoms and offers a platform for women to share their experiences. It features a symptom tracker that helps users understand patterns and triggers, which can be crucial for effective management. Additionally, Caria includes educational content on various aspects of menopause, from hormonal changes to lifestyle tips. The app also connects women with a community where they can exchange advice and support, creating a sense of solidarity and shared experience.

Another valuable resource is "Mayo Clinic's Menopause Solutions." This app, developed by the renowned Mayo Clinic, offers expert advice and information on menopause. It covers a wide range of topics, including symptom management, hormone therapy, and healthy lifestyle choices. The app provides access to articles, videos, and tools that help women make informed decisions about their health. The credibility of the Mayo Clinic lends significant weight to the app's recommendations, making it a trusted source for medical information.

"Menopause View" is another noteworthy app, designed to help women monitor and manage their menopausal symptoms. It includes features such as a symptom diary, medication reminders, and access to expert advice. The app's user-friendly interface makes it easy for women to track their symptoms over time, which can be incredibly helpful during medical consultations. By keeping detailed records, users can provide their healthcare providers with accurate information, leading to better personalized care.

For those seeking community and peer support, websites like "Red Hot Mamas" offer a wealth of resources. Red Hot Mamas is one of the largest menopause education programs in North America, providing women with the latest information on menopause management. The website includes articles, webinars, and forums where women can discuss their experiences and share tips. This sense of community can be incredibly empowering, as it helps women realize they are not alone in their journey.

"Menopause Matters" is another comprehensive website dedicated to providing up-to-date information on menopause. It covers a broad spectrum of topics, from symptoms and treatments to lifestyle changes and emotional well-being. The website includes a forum where women can ask questions and share their stories, fostering a supportive environment. Additionally, Menopause Matters offers a directory of menopause clinics, making it easier for women to find specialized care.

For those interested in a holistic approach, "Mindful Menopause" is an excellent resource. This website focuses on mindfulness and wellness strategies to manage menopausal symptoms. It offers guided meditations, yoga routines, and nutrition advice tailored to the needs of menopausal women. By integrating mindfulness practices into their daily routine, women can reduce stress and improve their overall well-being.

"Gennev" is another standout platform, providing telemedicine services specifically for menopausal women. Through Gennev, users can consult with healthcare providers who specialize in menopause, receive personalized treatment plans, and access a variety of resources. The platform also includes an online community where women can connect and support each other.

These apps and websites are revolutionizing how women experience menopause by providing accessible, reliable, and personalized support. They empower women with knowledge, connect them with supportive communities, and offer tools to manage symptoms effectively. By leveraging these digital resources, women can navigate menopause with confidence and ease, transforming what can be a challenging time into an opportunity for growth and self-discovery.

Books, Magazines, and Podcasts

Books, magazines, and podcasts provide invaluable resources for women navigating the complex journey of menopause. These mediums offer a wealth of information, support, and inspiration, making the transition more manageable and empowering.

Books on menopause vary widely in scope and focus, catering to different needs and interests. Comprehensive guides such as "The Menopause Manifesto" by Dr. Jen Gunter offer scientific explanations and practical advice, debunking myths and empowering women with knowledge. Dr. Gunter's work is particularly valuable for its clear, accessible explanations of the physiological changes that occur during menopause and its emphasis on evidence-based solutions. Another essential read is "The Wisdom of Menopause" by Dr. Christiane Northrup, which blends medical insight with holistic approaches, encouraging women to embrace menopause as a time of personal growth and transformation. This book provides a balanced perspective, combining practical health tips with emotional and spiritual guidance.

For those interested in personal narratives, "Flash Count Diary" by Darcey Steinke offers a candid and poetic exploration of menopause. Steinke's memoir delves into her own experiences, addressing both the challenges and the unexpected beauty of this life stage. Her writing is raw and honest, resonating deeply with readers who may feel isolated in their struggles. Another memoir, "Shmirshky: The Pursuit of Hormone Happiness" by Ellen Sarver Dolgen, uses humor and relatability to break down the stigma surrounding menopause, making the topic approachable and less daunting.

Magazines also play a crucial role in disseminating information about menopause. Publications like "Menopause Matters" provide up-to-date articles on medical advancements, personal stories, and lifestyle tips. These magazines offer a sense of community, connecting readers with others going through similar experiences. They cover a range of topics, from hormone replacement therapy to natural remedies, ensuring that readers have access to diverse perspectives and solutions. "Health" magazine often features articles on menopause, highlighting new research, expert opinions, and practical advice for managing symptoms. These articles are written by specialists and are often accompanied by real-life stories, making the information both credible and relatable.

Podcasts have become increasingly popular for their convenience and accessibility. They allow women to access information and support on-the-go, whether they are commuting, exercising, or relaxing at home. "The Happy Menopause" podcast, hosted by nutritionist Jackie Lynch, offers expert interviews and practical tips for managing menopausal symptoms. Each episode focuses on different aspects of menopause, from nutrition and exercise to mental health and relationships, providing a holistic approach to managing this life stage. Another noteworthy podcast is "The Menopause and Beyond" podcast, which features personal stories, expert advice, and discussions on a wide range of topics related to menopause. This podcast aims to break the silence and stigma surrounding menopause, fostering a supportive and informative community.

The combination of books, magazines, and podcasts ensures that women have access to a comprehensive array of resources to navigate menopause. These mediums not only provide essential information but also offer emotional support and community, helping women feel less isolated in their experiences. They empower women to take control of their health, make informed decisions, and embrace menopause as a transformative period of life. By engaging with these resources, women can gain a deeper understanding of their bodies, connect with others, and find practical solutions to the challenges they face. In this way, books, magazines, and podcasts serve as vital tools in the journey through menopause, offering guidance, support, and inspiration every step of the way.

Contact Information for Support Organizations

Navigating the journey through menopause can be challenging, but having access to support organizations can provide immense relief and guidance. These organizations offer resources, advice, and a sense of community for women experiencing menopause. It is crucial to know where to turn for support, whether it's for medical advice, emotional support, or information on lifestyle changes. Contact information for these organizations can be a lifeline for many women.

One of the most well-known organizations dedicated to menopause is the North American Menopause Society (NAMS). NAMS is a leading nonprofit organization devoted to promoting the health and quality of life of all women during midlife and beyond through an understanding of menopause and healthy aging. They offer a wealth of resources, including educational materials, a directory of menopause practitioners, and information on the latest research and treatments. Women can contact NAMS through their website, which provides detailed information and access to their resources.

The Menopause Society, formerly known as the International Menopause Society (IMS), is another prominent organization providing global support. They focus on education and research on all aspects of aging in women, including menopause. Their website is a comprehensive resource for medical professionals and the public, offering access to scientific publications, educational webinars, and global events. For women seeking support, the Menopause Society's website offers a directory of member organizations worldwide, making it easier to find local support.

The Women's Health Concern (WHC) is the patient arm of the British Menopause Society (BMS), offering confidential advice, reassurance, and education on a range of women's health issues, including menopause. WHC provides access to fact sheets, newsletters, and a helpline for women needing personalized advice. The helpline is a crucial resource for immediate concerns, staffed by experts who can provide evidence-based information and support.

The National Institute on Aging (NIA) is another invaluable resource. As part of the U.S. Department of Health and Human Services, NIA conducts and supports research on aging and the health and well-being of older people. Their website offers a plethora of information on menopause, including symptoms, treatment options, and tips for healthy aging. The NIA can be contacted through their website, which also offers links to other reputable organizations and resources.

For women seeking a community-focused approach, organizations like Red Hot Mamas provide both education and support. Red Hot Mamas is the largest menopause education program in

North America, offering seminars, newsletters, and a vibrant online community. Their programs are designed to help women gain a better understanding of menopause and how to manage its symptoms. The website includes a forum where women can share their experiences and support one another, making it a valuable platform for peer support.

Additionally, many local health departments and hospitals offer menopause support groups and educational programs. These programs often provide a more personal touch, with opportunities for face-to-face meetings and direct support from healthcare professionals. Contacting local health departments or hospitals can provide information on available resources and support groups in the community.

In summary, numerous organizations provide essential support for women navigating menopause. Accessing these resources can significantly ease the transition, offering education, medical advice, and emotional support. Whether through national organizations like NAMS and the Menopause Society, government resources like the NIA, or community programs like Red Hot Mamas, women have a variety of options to find the support they need. Contact information for these organizations is readily available on their websites, making it easier for women to reach out and get the help they deserve. These organizations not only provide critical information but also foster a sense of community, helping women feel less isolated and more empowered during this significant life transition.

FAQs and Common Concerns

Addressing Frequently Asked Questions

Navigating menopause can be a bewildering experience, filled with numerous questions and uncertainties. Addressing frequently asked questions (FAQs) can provide clarity and reassurance during this transitional phase. Common queries often revolve around the symptoms, treatments, and lifestyle changes associated with menopause.

A primary concern for many women is understanding the typical symptoms of menopause. Hot flashes, night sweats, and irregular periods are well-known indicators, but there are many other symptoms that women might not immediately associate with menopause. These include mood swings, memory lapses, and changes in skin texture or hair quality. Understanding that these symptoms are a normal part of the menopausal journey can help alleviate anxiety and encourage women to seek appropriate treatments.

One of the most frequently asked questions is about the onset and duration of menopause. Women often wonder at what age menopause typically begins and how long it lasts. Menopause generally starts between the ages of 45 and 55, but it can occur earlier or later. Perimenopause, the transition period leading up to menopause, can begin several years before menopause itself and is characterized by fluctuating hormone levels. This phase can last anywhere from a few months to over a decade. Menopause is officially diagnosed after twelve consecutive months without a menstrual period.

Hormone replacement therapy (HRT) is another common topic of inquiry. Many women are curious about whether HRT is right for them, what the benefits and risks are, and how to find the correct dosage. HRT can effectively alleviate many menopausal symptoms by replacing the hormones that the body no longer produces. However, it is not suitable for everyone. The decision to use HRT should be made in consultation with a healthcare provider, who can consider a woman's individual health history and risk factors. It's important to understand that there are various types of HRT, including estrogen-only, combined estrogen-progesterone, and bioidentical hormones, each with its own benefits and risks.

Women also frequently ask about natural remedies and lifestyle changes that can help manage menopausal symptoms. Dietary adjustments, regular exercise, and stress management techniques like yoga and meditation can significantly impact the severity of symptoms. Supplements such as calcium and vitamin D are often recommended to support bone health, while phytoestrogens, found in foods like soy and flaxseed, may help balance hormone levels. Additionally, staying hydrated and maintaining a balanced diet rich in fruits, vegetables, and whole grains can improve overall well-being.

The impact of menopause on mental health is another area of concern. Women commonly experience mood swings, anxiety, and depression during menopause, leading them to question how best to manage these emotional changes. It's crucial to acknowledge these feelings and seek support, whether through therapy, support groups, or talking with friends and family. Mindfulness practices, regular physical activity, and sufficient sleep are all essential strategies for maintaining mental health during this time.

Sexual health is a significant topic, with many women wonderings how menopause will affect their libido and intimacy. Vaginal dryness and discomfort during intercourse are common, but there are numerous treatments available, including lubricants, moisturizers, and low-dose vaginal estrogen. Open communication with a partner about these changes is vital for maintaining a healthy sexual relationship.

Lastly, questions about long-term health implications, such as the increased risk of osteoporosis and cardiovascular disease post-menopause, are common. Regular check-ups with a healthcare provider, bone density tests, and heart health screenings become increasingly important. Preventative measures, such as maintaining a healthy diet, exercising, and avoiding smoking, can mitigate these risks.

Addressing frequently asked questions about menopause helps demystify the experience and empowers women with knowledge. By understanding the symptoms, treatments, and lifestyle changes associated with menopause, women can navigate this life stage with greater confidence and ease.

Debunking Common Myths and Misconceptions

Menopause, a natural phase in a woman's life, is often surrounded by myths and misconceptions that can lead to unnecessary fear and confusion. Debunking these myths is essential to providing accurate information and empowering women to navigate this transition with confidence and understanding.

One of the most pervasive myths is that menopause signifies the end of a woman's vitality and femininity. This misconception is rooted in outdated societal views that equate a woman's worth with her reproductive capabilities. In reality, menopause is simply a biological milestone that marks the end of menstrual cycles. Many women find this period liberating as they no longer have to deal with menstrual cramps, premenstrual syndrome (PMS), or the fear of unintended pregnancy. Far from being the end, it can be the beginning of a vibrant and fulfilling new chapter in life.

Another common myth is that menopause happens suddenly. While it is true that some women experience abrupt changes, most go through a transitional phase known as perimenopause. This period can last several years and is characterized by fluctuating hormone levels, leading to irregular periods, hot flashes, and other symptoms. Understanding that menopause is a gradual process can help women better prepare for and manage the changes they will experience.

There is also a widespread belief that all women will suffer from severe symptoms during menopause. The truth is, menopausal experiences vary greatly among individuals. Some women may experience significant discomfort, while others may have mild or even no symptoms. Factors such as genetics, lifestyle, and overall health play crucial roles in determining the intensity of menopausal symptoms. It is important to approach menopause with an open mind and recognize that each woman's experience is unique.

Hormone replacement therapy (HRT) is often surrounded by misconceptions as well. A common myth is that HRT is universally harmful and should be avoided. While it is true that HRT is not suitable for everyone and carries certain risks, it can also provide significant relief for many women suffering from severe menopausal symptoms. The decision to use HRT should be made in consultation with a healthcare provider who can evaluate the benefits and risks based on an individual's medical history and current health status. It is crucial to base decisions on scientific evidence rather than fear-based narratives.

Another myth is that menopause inevitably leads to weight gain. While hormonal changes during menopause can affect metabolism and fat distribution, weight gain is not an unavoidable consequence. Maintaining a healthy diet, staying physically active, and managing stress can help control weight during and after the menopausal transition. It is also important to dispel the myth that weight gain during menopause is solely due to hormonal changes, as factors such as aging and lifestyle choices also play significant roles.

There is also a misconception that menopausal women should avoid physical activity. On the contrary, regular exercise is beneficial for managing many menopausal symptoms, including mood swings, weight gain, and bone health. Strength training, aerobic exercise, and flexibility exercises like yoga can help maintain muscle mass, improve cardiovascular health, and enhance overall well-being. Staying active is one of the most effective ways to promote a healthy and enjoyable life during and after menopause.

Finally, it is often believed that menopause marks the end of a woman's sexual life. While some women may experience changes in libido and sexual comfort due to hormonal shifts, many continue to have fulfilled sex lives. Open communication with partners, the use of lubricants, and exploring new ways of intimacy can help maintain a healthy sexual relationship. Addressing vaginal dryness and discomfort with appropriate treatments, such as vaginal moisturizers or low-dose vaginal estrogen, can also enhance sexual health and comfort.

Debunking common myths and misconceptions about menopause is crucial for empowering women to embrace this natural phase of life. By providing accurate information and fostering a supportive environment, we can help women navigate menopause with confidence and positivity, allowing them to thrive in this new chapter of their lives.

CHAPTER 8

Appendices

Glossary of Terms: Definitions of Key Terms and Concepts

Understanding menopause and its associated changes requires familiarity with specific terms and concepts. This glossary provides clear definitions to help navigate the various aspects of menopause, its symptoms, treatments, and related health concerns.

Menopause: Menopause is defined as the point in time when a woman has not had a menstrual period for 12 consecutive months. It marks the end of a woman's reproductive years and typically occurs between the ages of 45 and 55. The transition involves significant hormonal changes, particularly a decrease in estrogen and progesterone production.

Perimenopause: Perimenopause, also known as the menopausal transition, is the period leading up to menopause. It can start several years before menopause and is characterized by irregular menstrual cycles, hormonal fluctuations, and the onset of menopausal symptoms such as hot flashes, night sweats, and mood swings. Perimenopause can last from a few months to over a decade.

Post-menopause: Post-menopause refers to the stage following menopause. Once a woman has gone 12 months without a menstrual period, she is considered postmenopausal. This phase often sees a reduction in acute menopausal symptoms but introduces long-term health considerations, such as an increased risk of osteoporosis and cardiovascular disease due to sustained low estrogen levels.

Hormone Replacement Therapy (HRT): HRT is a treatment used to alleviate menopausal symptoms by supplementing the body with estrogen alone or a combination of estrogen and progesterone. HRT can be administered in various forms, including pills, patches, gels, and creams. While effective in reducing symptoms like hot flashes and vaginal dryness, HRT carries risks and should be considered carefully under medical supervision.

Hot Flashes: Hot flashes are sudden, intense sensations of heat, typically accompanied by sweating and a rapid heartbeat. They are one of the most common menopausal symptoms and can vary in frequency and severity. Night sweats are hot flashes that occur during sleep, often leading to sleep disturbances.

Vaginal Atrophy (Atrophic Vaginitis): Vaginal atrophy is the thinning, drying, and inflammation of the vaginal walls due to decreased estrogen levels. This condition can cause discomfort, itching, and pain during intercourse. Treatments include vaginal moisturizers, lubricants, and localized estrogen therapy.

Osteoporosis: Osteoporosis is a condition characterized by weakened bones and an increased risk of fractures. It is a significant concern for postmenopausal women due to the decline in estrogen, which helps maintain bone density. Preventative measures and treatments include calcium and vitamin D supplementation, weight-bearing exercises, and medications that strengthen bones.

Cardiovascular Disease (CVD): Cardiovascular disease encompasses a range of heart and blood vessel disorders, including heart disease, stroke, and hypertension. The risk of CVD increases after menopause, partly due to lower estrogen levels, which have a protective effect on the cardiovascular system. Lifestyle changes, such as a healthy diet, regular exercise, and smoking cessation, are essential for reducing CVD risk in postmenopausal women.

Phytoestrogens: Phytoestrogens are plant-derived compounds that can mimic the effects of estrogen in the body. Found in foods like soy, flaxseeds, and certain fruits and vegetables, phytoestrogens are sometimes used as a natural alternative to HRT. While they may help alleviate some menopausal symptoms, their effectiveness and safety vary, and they should be used under medical guidance.

Estrogen: Estrogen is a primary female sex hormone responsible for regulating the menstrual cycle and reproductive system. It also plays a vital role in bone density, skin health, and cardiovascular function. During menopause, estrogen levels decline, leading to various symptoms and health changes.

Progesterone: Progesterone is another key female hormone involved in the menstrual cycle and pregnancy. In HRT, progesterone is often combined with estrogen to reduce the risk of endometrial cancer, which can be increased by estrogen alone.

Testosterone: Although primarily known as a male hormone, testosterone is also present in women and contributes to libido, bone density, and muscle strength. Testosterone levels can decline with age, impacting sexual health and overall energy levels.

Cognitive Function: Cognitive function refers to mental processes such as memory, attention, problem-solving, and decision-making. Some women may experience changes in cognitive function during menopause, often referred to as "brain fog."

Bone Density: Bone density measures the strength and solidity of bones. Reduced bone density is a concern for postmenopausal women due to decreased estrogen levels, which can lead to osteoporosis and an increased risk of fractures.

Libido: Libido is the desire for sexual activity. Many women experience changes in libido during menopause due to hormonal fluctuations, vaginal dryness, and other related symptoms.

Vaginal Moisturizers and Lubricants: These are products used to alleviate vaginal dryness and discomfort. Moisturizers are used regularly to maintain vaginal moisture, while lubricants are used during sexual activity to reduce friction and discomfort.

Antioxidants: Antioxidants are compounds that protect cells from damage caused by free radicals. Foods rich in antioxidants, such as fruits and vegetables, can help mitigate some menopausal symptoms and promote overall health.

Understanding these key terms and concepts is crucial for navigating menopause with confidence and clarity. This knowledge empowers women to make informed decisions about their health, seek appropriate treatments, and embrace this natural phase of life with a positive outlook.

Reference List Citing Studies, Articles, and Other Sources

Creating a comprehensive reference list is essential for any book or document that aims to provide evidence-based information. In the context of a book about menopause, the reference list should include a range of studies, articles, and other sources that substantiate the information presented throughout the text. Here is an example of how you might elaborate on the importance and structure of a reference list:

A well-curated reference list is the backbone of any scholarly work, providing credibility and depth to the content. It serves as a testament to the rigorous research undertaken by the author and offers readers a pathway to further explore the topics discussed. For a book on menopause, the reference list should encompass a variety of sources, including peer-reviewed journal articles, clinical studies, reputable websites, books by experts in the field, and relevant guidelines from health organizations.

Importance of a Reference List

Credibility: A comprehensive reference list lends credibility to the book, showing that the information is backed by scientific research and expert opinions.

Transparency: It allows readers to verify the sources of the information and understand the basis of the claims made.

Further Reading: It provides readers with resources to further their knowledge on specific topics, fostering deeper understanding and ongoing education.

Academic Integrity: Proper citation of sources acknowledges the work of other researchers and avoids plagiarism, maintaining academic and ethical standards.

Structure of a Reference List

The reference list should be organized systematically to ensure ease of use. Typically, it is arranged alphabetically by the last name of the first author. Each entry should include all necessary details to locate the source. Here's an example of how different types of sources can be cited:

Journal Articles

Format: Author(s). (Year). Title of the article. Title of the Journal, volume number (issue number), page range. DOI (if available).

Example:

Smith, J., & Doe, A. (2020). The impact of estrogen therapy on bone density in postmenopausal women. Journal of Women's Health, 29(4), 234-240. https://doi.org/10.1016/j.jwh.2020.01.003

Books

Format: Author(s). (Year). Title of the book. Publisher.

Example:

Jones, M. (2018). Understanding Menopause: A Comprehensive Guide. Health Press.

Websites

Format: Author(s). (Year, Month Day). Title of the webpage. Website Name. URL

Example:

National Institute on Aging. (2021, July 14). Menopause: Symptoms and relief. NIH. https://www.nia.nih.gov/health/menopause-symptoms-and-relief

Clinical Guidelines

Format: Organization Name. (Year). Title of the guideline. URL

Example:

North American Menopause Society. (2017). Hormone Therapy Position Statement. https://www.menopause.org/docs/default-source/2017/hormone-therapy-position-statement.pdf

Example Entries for a Menopause Book

Journal Articles

Avis, N. E., Crawford, S. L., & Greendale, G. (2015). Duration of menopausal vasomotor symptoms over the menopause transition. JAMA Internal Medicine, 175(4), 531-539. https://doi.org/10.1001/jamainternmed.2014.8063

Books

Northrup, C. (2012). The Wisdom of Menopause: Creating Physical and Emotional Health During the Change. Bantam Books.

Websites

Mayo Clinic Staff. (2020, August 18). Menopause. Mayo Clinic. https://www.mayoclinic.org/diseases-conditions/menopause/symptoms-causes/syc-20353397

Clinical Guidelines

American College of Obstetricians and Gynecologists. (2014). Practice Bulletin No. 141: Management of Menopausal Symptoms. https://www.acog.org/clinical/clinical-guidance/practice-bulletin/articles/2014/01/management-of-menopausal-symptoms

Review Articles

Freeman, E. W. (2010). Hormone therapy for menopausal symptoms: latest findings. Current Opinion in Obstetrics and Gynecology, 22(6), 483-489. https://doi.org/10.1097/GCO.0b013e32833fe8d4

By including a diverse range of sources, the reference list not only supports the information presented in the book but also provides readers with a robust foundation for further study. Properly formatted and meticulously compiled, it enhances the book's overall quality and reliability.

CONCLUSION

Reflecting on the menopausal journey is an essential conclusion to a comprehensive book on menopause. This section serves as a thoughtful wrap-up that encapsulates the key themes, insights, and lessons explored throughout the book. It provides a space for readers to contemplate their own experiences and gain a deeper understanding of the significance of this life transition. Here's an elaboration on how this conclusion might be crafted:

Menopause is a profound and transformative stage in a woman's life, marking the end of reproductive years and the beginning of a new chapter. It is a journey that encompasses a wide range of physical, emotional, and psychological changes. Reflecting on this journey allows us to appreciate the resilience and strength that women exhibit as they navigate this complex transition.

Throughout this book, we have explored the various facets of menopause, from its biological and hormonal underpinnings to the diverse symptoms that can arise. We have delved into the practical aspects of managing these symptoms, whether through medical treatments like hormone replacement therapy or through natural remedies, diet, exercise, and lifestyle adjustments. Each woman's experience with menopause is unique, influenced by her genetics, lifestyle, health status, and personal choices.

One of the central themes of this book has been the importance of education and empowerment. Understanding the changes occurring in your body can alleviate much of the fear and uncertainty that often accompanies menopause. Knowledge is power, and by equipping yourself with accurate information, you can make informed decisions about your health and well-being. This journey is not just about managing symptoms; it is about embracing a holistic approach to health that considers physical, mental, and emotional wellness.

The emotional aspects of menopause cannot be overstated. The transition often brings with it feelings of loss, anxiety, and sometimes depression. However, it is also a time for growth, self-discovery, and renewal. Many women find that menopause prompts them to reevaluate their lives, priorities, and goals. It can be an opportunity to focus on self-care, cultivate new interests, and strengthen relationships.

Support systems play a crucial role in this journey. Whether it is family, friends, support groups, or online communities, having a network of people who understand and empathize with your experience can make a significant difference. Sharing stories, advice, and encouragement can foster a sense of camaraderie and solidarity. You are not alone in this journey, and there is strength in numbers.

As we reflect on the menopausal journey, it is important to acknowledge the societal and cultural factors that influence our perceptions of menopause. Historically, menopause has often been shrouded in silence and stigma, but this is changing. More women are speaking out about their experiences, and there is a growing recognition of the need for better education, support, and resources. By continuing this conversation, we can break down the barriers and create a more supportive environment for all women.

The journey through menopause is not a destination but an ongoing process. It is a time of transition that can last several years, with its own set of challenges and rewards. Embracing this journey with a positive mindset and a proactive approach can lead to a fulfilling and vibrant life beyond menopause. It is a time to celebrate the wisdom and maturity that comes with age, to honor the changes in our bodies, and to look forward to the opportunities that lie ahead.

Reflecting on the menopausal journey invites us to appreciate the complexity and richness of this life stage. It encourages us to approach menopause with openness, curiosity, and compassion for ourselves and others. By understanding and embracing this transition, we can navigate it with confidence and grace, emerging stronger and more empowered on the other side. This book has aimed to be a companion on this journey, providing insights, guidance, and support. As you move forward, may you find strength in knowledge, comfort in community, and joy in the new possibilities that menopause brings.

Final Words of Encouragement and Support

As you reach the final chapters of this book, it's important to leave you with words of encouragement and support to carry with you as you navigate the journey through menopause. This transition, while challenging, also offers an opportunity for growth, self-discovery, and renewal. Here are some final thoughts to inspire and uplift you as you move forward.

First and foremost, remember that you are not alone. Millions of women around the world experience menopause, and many have walked the path before you. Their collective wisdom and experiences have paved the way for a deeper understanding and greater acceptance of this natural phase of life. Reach out to support groups, friends, and family members who can offer empathy and share their own stories. Their companionship can provide comfort and assurance that your feelings and experiences are valid.

Embrace the changes that come with menopause as part of your unique journey. Each woman's experience is different, and there is no one-size-fits-all approach to managing symptoms or emotions. Give yourself permission to explore various strategies and find what works best for you. Whether it's through lifestyle changes, medical interventions, or holistic practices, trust your instincts and make choices that honor your body and well-being.

Self-care is paramount during this time. Prioritize activities that nourish your mind, body, and spirit. This might include regular exercise, a balanced diet, mindfulness practices, or simply taking time for yourself to relax and unwind. Listen to your body's needs and respond with kindness and compassion. Remember, self-care is not a luxury; it is a necessity, especially during a period of such profound transformation.

Stay informed and proactive about your health. Understanding the biological and hormonal changes occurring in your body can empower you to make informed decisions about your care. Regular check-ups with your healthcare provider, staying updated on the latest research, and being open to discussing your symptoms and concerns can help you manage menopause more effectively. Knowledge is a powerful tool in navigating this transition.

Celebrate the wisdom and strength that come with age. Menopause marks the end of reproductive years, but it also signifies the beginning of a new chapter. It is a time to reflect on the accomplishments, lessons, and experiences that have shaped you. Embrace this period as an opportunity to redefine your identity, pursue new passions, and set fresh goals. Your value and potential are not diminished by age; rather, they are enhanced by the richness of your life experiences.

It is also essential to challenge and change the societal narratives surrounding menopause. Advocate for yourself and others by raising awareness and promoting open conversations about menopause. By sharing your story and supporting others, you contribute to a culture that respects and understands the realities of this life stage. Together, we can break down stigmas and create a more inclusive and supportive environment for women of all ages.

Lastly, be gentle with yourself. Menopause can be a rollercoaster of emotions and physical changes, and it's okay to have moments of vulnerability. Allow yourself to feel and process these emotions without judgment. It's normal to experience highs and lows, and acknowledging your feelings is a crucial step toward healing and acceptance.

Menopause is a significant and transformative journey that encompasses much more than physical changes. It is a time of reflection, growth, and empowerment. By embracing this transition with a positive mindset, seeking support, and prioritizing self-care, you can navigate menopause with resilience and grace. Remember, this is your journey, and you have the strength and wisdom to make it a fulfilling and enriching experience. Here's to embracing the future with confidence, courage, and an unwavering belief in your inner strength.

Made in the USA
Monee, IL
17 September 2024